INTEGRAL PSYCHOLOGY

SUNY series in Transpersonal and Humanistic Psychology
Richard D. Mann, editor

Integral Psychology

Yoga, Growth, and Opening the Heart

Brant Cortright

STATE UNIVERSITY OF NEW YORK PRESS

Published by
State University of New York Press, Albany

© 2007 State University of New York

Printed in the United States of America

For information, contact State University of New York Press, Albany, NY
www.sunypress.edu

Production by Michael Haggett
Marketing by Fran Keneston

Library of Congress Cataloging in Publication Data

Cortright, Brant, 1949–
    Integral psychology : yoga, growth, and opening the heart /
Brant Cortright.
        p. ; cm. — (SUNY series in transpersonal and humanistic psychology)
    Includes bibliographical references and index.
    ISBN-13: 978-0-7914-7071-8 (hardcover : alk. paper)
    ISBN-13: 978-0-7914-7072-5 (pbk. : alk. paper)
    1. Psychotherapy—Philosophy. 2. Holistic medicine. I. Title.
II. Series
    [DNLM: 1. Psychotherapy. 2. Holistic Health. 3. Mind-Body Relations
(Metaphysics) 4. Spirituality. 5. Yoga—psychology.
WM 420 C831i 2007]
RC437.5.C67 2007
616.89'14—dc22

                                                            2006016538

10 9 8 7 6 5 4 3 2 1

Dedicated to the Divine Shakti,
Mother of the Universe

Contents

Acknowledgments

I would like to thank many helpful friends, colleagues, students, and clients for their impact in shaping this book. Paul Herman first invited me to co-teach a course on Integral Psychology with him some 20 years ago, which eventually evolved into a course I currently teach yearly at the California Institute of Integral Studies. Paul's support at an early phase of my involvement in integral yoga was important to my continuing to work in this field. I am eternally grateful for this early collaboration.

Many colleagues, friends, and former students have read chapters of this manuscript and provided both critical feedback and encouragement. Among these are Michael Kahn, Robert McDermott, Brendan Collins, Bahman Shirazi, Richard Stein, Bryan Wittine, Paul Linn, Olga Louchakova, Matthijs Cornelissen, Neeltje Huppes, Ananda Reddy, Aster Patel, Uma Silbey, Kathleen Wall, and Nicolo Santilli. Mytrae Meliana read the entire manuscript and gave invaluable feedback that greatly enhanced the final result.

The staff at SUNY Press has been extremely helpful and highly professional. I want to thank Jane Bunker, Editor-in-Chief, for her guidance in this project and Michael Haggett for his precise and helpful editing.

I am deeply grateful to all.

Introduction

Oh, East is East, and West is West, and never the twain shall meet.
—Rudyard Kipling, *The Sayings of Rudyard Kipling*

Eastern and Western visions of psychology have lived in different worlds until recently. While they have begun to touch and even have some influence on each other, a wider synthesis has not yet occurred. In part, this is because Western psychological systems tend to be separative, dividing into competing schools and theories, and because spiritual systems also separate along a great divide, with seemingly mutually exclusive approaches to Spirit. Integrating the many streams of spirituality in a way that does not privilege one over the others has so far been elusive.

This book attempts a far-reaching integration of the East's and West's rich diversity of psychological thought. It brings together many things—East and West, body and mind, spirituality and psychology—to create an integral psychology and psychotherapy. It grows out of several decades of involvement in both Eastern and Western psychology and more than 20 years' immersion in Sri Aurobindo's integral yoga. For much of this time, my interests in spirituality and psychology moved along parallel tracks. Synthesizing these two directions into a unifying vision took much time and experimentation, traveling in different directions that sometimes were fruitful but other times came to dead ends. My teaching at the California Institute of Integral Studies has been crucial in integrating these two dimensions of human existence.

The integral yoga and integral philosophy of Sri Aurobindo is a gold mine of spiritual and psychological wisdom. What is hard to understand is why his philosophy is not better known, not only in the West but in India as well. While efforts have been made to popularize his writings, using philosophy as the medium for this has not yielded

1

notable results thus far. My own hope is that this may happen through psychology, and this book charts some first steps toward an integral approach to healing, growth, and transformation.

A BRIEF DIGRESSION INTO THE SPIRITUAL CONTEXT

(*Note:* At this point, the interested reader is encouraged to read a fuller account provided in appendix A.)

All psychological systems arise within a particular spiritual and philosophical context and construct their view of the human being from basic assumptions embedded in this context. Whether this philosophical context is materialistic or spiritual has profound implications for the psychology that emerges. The field of psychology was born and grew up in a materialistic atmosphere. Freud, the founder of modern depth psychology, was adamantly atheistic, and his theories and most of those that followed him reflected this bias. Academic psychology, attempting to mimic the natural sciences in its early years, also excluded spirituality from research and hewed to a purely empirical, materialistic paradigm.

This book presupposes that it is better to explicitly examine the spiritual context than to suffer the consequences of unexamined, implicit assumptions in our psychological systems. In a materialistic philosophy that holds biology to be ultimate, psychologies that proceed from this assumption lead to certain conclusions about consciousness, behavior, and the possibilities for human growth. Even the idea of healing, of what is possible and how far it can go, is skewed by this context, for the healing force is seen to be entirely physical rather than spiritual, and this severely limits the possibilities that can be envisioned. On the other hand, when our spiritual nature is affirmed as the foundation of human consciousness, the psychologies that emerge from this view are radically different in how they view the psyche and its potentials. The greatest thinkers from the religious traditions of the world are unanimous in their verdict that failing to see the spiritual dimension of human consciousness as fundamental leads to limited and ultimately incorrect psychologies.

Informed by a postmodern sensibility that acknowledges the historical, cultural, and linguistic contexts operative in the construction of all knowledge, psychology has been undergoing a quiet revolution.

Knowledge, according to postmodern thinking, can be constructed from infinite perspectives, and therefore there must be a plurality of viewpoints that have truth value. Here postmodernism and Eastern spiritual systems coincide. They come to the same fundamental position, namely, that *the human mind can never know Truth*. Mental knowing is inherently perspectival and partial, so it is incapable of truth unalloyed.

This is precisely what the East has said for more than 2,000 years: Ultimate truth is beyond the mind's grasp. The futility of mind's attempt to grasp truth is an astonishing point of agreement between ancient traditions and postmodernism.

However, here postmodernism continues on and makes another, entirely unjustified assertion: *Therefore, there is no ultimate truth.* Postmodernism leaps beyond its own recognized limits to assert a claim that it has just conceded cannot be made, an observation made by several commentators but that has not yet corrected the problem (e.g., see Smith, 1982.) It is a seductive leap, yet a strictly postmodern position can only be agnostic on the question of ultimate truth.

While postmodernism helpfully shows how personal perspective shapes the construction of knowledge, postmodernism, by its incapacity to penetrate beyond surface appearances, does psychology a disservice in denying all deeper realities and essentialist claims to truth. All psychologies rooted in postmodernism will thus be psychologies of the surface, helpful so far as they go but confined to a view of frontal appearances. A unifying view of psychology therefore requires a more encompassing perspective.

Here Eastern psychology comes to the rescue. The Eastern traditions declare that there *is* an essential truth, an essential spiritual reality that is known by many names, imaged in many forms, including formlessness, represented by the mind in infinite ways yet beyond all concepts and formulations. To go beyond the surface mind and experience this deeper reality is the goal of Eastern practices. When the goal is wholeness, only methodologies that go beyond the mind's fragmentary approaches can comprehend this wholeness.

When Swami Vivekananda first brought Hinduism to the West at the dawn of the 20th century, he correctly proclaimed Vedanta India's most precious gift to the world. Hinduism is one world religion that does not originate from the experiences of a single man. Instead, it is the combined wisdom of many centuries of sages and saints who have explored the inner realms of consciousness from a thousand different directions. This work draws on the psychological discoveries of Vedanta, particularly the integral Vedanta of Sri Aurobindo, a culminating figure in India's philosophical history who made a highly sophisticated integration of the major systems of Indian philosophy.

The world's spiritual traditions tend to fall into two broad classes: theism, or the vision of the Divine as a Personal, Supreme Being, and nontheism, or the vision of the Divine as an Impersonal, infinite consciousness. Viewing the Divine as both Personal and Impersonal corresponds to our dual spiritual identity—soul and spirit, also called *antaratman* and atman, or psychic center and Buddha-nature.

Integral yoga philosophy puts spirituality into an evolutionary context. Life is a divine unfolding, and the foundation is *sat-chit-ananda* (i.e., the Divine is a self-existent, blissful consciousness). The Divine throws itself into form to create this entire universe as a play of self-discovery. Out of matter evolves life, out of life evolves mind, and now with these evolved instruments, spirit is emerging in physical form. However, it takes time for consciousness to evolve. Consciousness does not spring fully into being or leap miraculously from an insect to an enlightened sage. It undergoes a systematic growth, a developmental process of ever-increasing power, amplitude, depth, and capacity. Since it is a gradual, incremental development of consciousness that is occurring over great spans of time, this requires a number of different physical forms within which to evolve, so reincarnation becomes a logical and practical necessity, with birth and death as incidents or transitions in the soul's growth.

The purpose is a joyous and conscious participation in the evolutionary play, not a withdrawal from life, not fleeing embodied existence into a heaven or nirvana. Existence is not viewed as a mistake or a cosmic nightmare from which we need to escape. Integral philosophy is life affirming, not life negating, like the doctrine of illusionism (or *mayavada*), which had such a destructive effect on India and much of the East. The Divine is not seeking to annul its own creation. Life is real, not merely an illusion, though it is an ignorance in our current state. The goal is to wake up to our deeper identity so we can align with this larger, Divine movement of love and delight. Life is a spiritual adventure in the evolution of consciousness. Spiritual embodiment is the goal, not a disembodied transcendence. For this we need to discover our soul, our psychic center, which is the evolutionary principle in us.

Integral philosophy is an integrating framework for all the world's spiritual traditions—theistic and nontheistic, Eastern and Western. It includes all spiritual paths without privileging one over another. Every spiritual tradition is honored, for all lead to the one Divine (Brahman, God, Allah, Buddha-nature, Tao.)

There is a striking image in the Hindu tradition of a statue or picture of Shiva dancing. Twirling four arms, in perfect serenity and bliss, Shiva brings this world into manifestation through his dance. Shiva dances for the sheer bliss of dancing. There is no other motive or goal, just the pure joy of dancing. To see that the Divine, out of the fullness of self-expression and the utter delight of play, has manifested this entire universe gives a new appreciation for life's potential for delight and fulfillment.

THE DESIGN OF THIS BOOK

Two important terms are used throughout this book that are necessary to understand at the outset: *soul* and *integral*. "Soul" is used in so many ways today that it can be hard to know what is meant. Generally, soul means the deeper parts of the personality, or sometimes the mind or the mind and heart together. At other times it means the immortal, eternal soul of spiritual traditions. In this book, soul has the latter meaning, though with a unique understanding that the soul is an evolving entity. The soul is our inmost identity, our psychic center, and the evolutionary principle in human beings. It survives death and creates a new body-heart-mind complex each new lifetime through which it expresses itself.

The word "integral" is becoming popular these days, and there is understandable confusion about what it means. Integral has two basic meanings: large and narrow. In its larger, generic sense, integral means whole, complete, and holistic, and it can include such things as body-mind-spirit as well as East-West. This is the sense in which it is usually used by such people as Gerard (1988) and Wilber (2000.) The narrow meaning of integral comes from the integral yoga and integral philosophy of Sri Aurobindo, sometimes called India's greatest mystic philosopher. It was in this sense that an Indian psychologist, Indra Sen, first coined the term "integral psychology" in a series of professional papers in India throughout the 1930s, 40s, and 50s. Curiously, the

narrow meaning includes the larger meaning, although the large meaning does not include the narrow. It is this more specific sense of integral that is meant throughout this book—the integral psychology and
integral psychotherapy that emerges from the integral yoga of Sri
Aurobindo.

Part 1 of this book brings integrality to bear on psychology. Chapter 1 integrates Eastern and Western psychology's many voices into a
coherent whole. Chapter 2 brings out an immensely important discovery of integral psychology about the nature of the psyche that has never
been clearly seen by Western psychology. Chapter 3 explores how the
core wounding of our time has a clouding, obscuring effect on our
awareness of our deeper identity. Chapter 4 provides an integrative
vision of psychotherapy's potential and points toward new evolutionary
possibilities for psychological health.

Part 2 brings integrality to bear on psychotherapy practice, synthesizing Eastern and Western methods for discovering wholeness. Using
the lens of the three traditional yogas—*karma* yoga, *jnana* yoga, and
bhakti yoga—provides a way of organizing the methods of psychotherapy into an integral psycho-spiritual practice. The final chapter then
provides an integrative approach to psychotherapy.

Part 1

Integral Psychology

Chapter 1

Integrality

Psychology is the study of mind and behavior.
—American psychology textbook

Psychology is the science of consciousness.
—Sri Aurobindo, *Essays Divine
and Human*

This book aims to integrate two diverse streams of psychology: Western and Eastern. Each of these streams has made profound discoveries about the psyche, human consciousness, the nature of fragmentation, and the possibilities for wholeness. Yet psychology in the West and psychology in the East have traveled from two different directions and developed very different areas of knowledge. This chapter begins with a broad characterization of these two streams of psychological thought in order to highlight these differences.

Psychology in the West looks from the *outside in*, whereas psychology in the East looks from the *inside out*. These two perspectives give two very different views of psychology. By looking from the outside in, Western psychology has developed very detailed, precise maps of the outer being, the body-heart-mind organism and the self, whereas Eastern psychology's view from the inside out has generated very detailed maps of our inner being and the spiritual foundation of consciousness. Each has essential knowledge about human existence, yet each focuses on only half of this psycho-spiritual totality. Each requires the other to

9

complete it, and only in bringing them together does an integral view of psychology emerge.

Western psychology ascribes our lack of wholeness and painful fragmentation to the universal experience of psychological wounding. *We do not know the fullness of who we are because our wounding makes us unconscious of it.* While some people are wounded more severely and some less, we all are wounded. To be born into this world is to be emotionally hurt and scarred growing up. Our response to this wounding is to push it down, contract, and develop a defensive structure in which large portions of our very self become unconscious. We become lost, isolated from others, cut off and alienated from our own deeper self. Western psychotherapy is an attempt to understand and repair this fragmented wholeness.

Eastern psychology sees a different cause for our fragmentation and suffering: *We are cut off from the spiritual ground of our being.* We identify with the surface life of our body and ego—our desires, feelings, sensations, thoughts—and so are unconscious of our spiritual source. Eastern psychological practices aim at bringing peace and harmony into our living, so we may go deeply inside to find the true fulfillment intrinsic to our spiritual core.

The human predicament, then, is characterized by a double fragmentation. It is a dual diagnosis from which we suffer—a psycho-spiritual fracture—and dual, therefore, must be the path to wholeness.

THE QUEST FOR WHOLENESS

Every human being seeks a better life. Whether clearly experienced or only vaguely felt, there is a sense that something greater is possible. This search may take a superficial form such as striving to acquire money, position, or power; it may manifest as a yearning for fulfillment through relationships and love; or it may lie in seeking higher values such as meaning, peace, or helping others. But through all of this there is an intuitive feeling that what we seek lies beyond all these first reachings. For once beyond looking outward for this deeper fulfillment in things and people, we realize that it is an inner state we are seeking. This search, at bottom, is a quest for wholeness.

Western psychology seeks for wholeness in both theory and practice: in the search for a comprehensive understanding of human nature and in the search for methods to heal the wounded, divided self. Yet like the human being it attempts to understand, Western psychology itself is a field divided, fragmented into a bewildering array of competing theories and conflicting therapies that makes it seem more like a fractious and unruly mob than a well-ordered, consistent discipline. The current state of Western psychology resembles the biblical story of the Tower of Babel: Cognitive psychologists do not talk to body therapists. Psychoanalysts look down on gestalt therapists. Academic psychologists complain that clinicians are not scientific, and clinicians complain that academic researchers are superficial. Jungians do not send their children to schools run by behaviorists, and for their part, most behaviorists would not be caught dead talking to a Jungian about soul. Psychology as a whole is characterized both by the explosive growth of its many disparate fragments and its lack of an integrating structure that brings together the various factions into a coherent whole.

Further, a postmodern perspective raises the question of what becomes "knowledge" in psychology. Historically, what constitutes psychological knowledge has been narrowly Western and has excluded cultures in which the depth of psychological thought in significant ways surpasses the West. It must be conceded from the outset that while Western psychology has generated a great mass of detailed knowledge of the surface of the psyche, it has failed to penetrate its deeper mysteries, for even depth psychology is but a psychology of the frontal self and its unconscious processes. Western psychology has only explored the surface of consciousness, because its instruments of investigation are fragmentary and limited.

As science so often reminds us, real understanding comes when we look past the surface appearance of things into their deeper nature. Otherwise, for example, we are led to believe the initial view given by our senses, that the sun travels around the earth. Just as we need to look beyond first appearances in astronomy, physics, and other hard sciences, so we need to look deeply in psychology. As more sophisticated instruments have advanced the hard sciences—microscopes, telescopes, particle accelerators—so more sophisticated methods of consciousness exploration have allowed Eastern psychology to come upon a deeper, wider, more fundamental knowledge of the psyche than Western psychology.

To understand the depths of human consciousness, the instrument of exploration can only be consciousness itself. The West's "outside in" approach of external observations, brain imaging instruments such as MRIs, fMRIs, EEGs, PET scans, and so on, and even the surface introspective methods of depth psychotherapy, helpful as they are, will only take us so far. To bring about a more complete understanding, well-defined methods of inner exploration must be employed, and it is in this area that the Eastern meditative traditions excel, for Eastern spiritual systems are the result of centuries of rigorous, precise applications of methods for examining inner states of consciousness.

Eastern spiritual systems, and India in particular, have made a highly disciplined study of consciousness and the psyche for millennia. Although traditional Western psychology has relegated Eastern psychological thought to philosophy or religion, a current appraisal of psychology must include Eastern cultures' contributions to psychology. As globalization increases, the current Western-centric view of psychology (Cushman, 1995) is being counterbalanced by developments such as India's recent movement of "Indian psychology" (Cornelisson & Joshi, 2004), which seeks to re-own Indian psychological insights and situate them in their proper field of psychology, following Gardiner Murphy's pioneering work (Murphy, 1958.) From a global perspective, a strictly Western definition of psychology that excludes the East's profound discoveries appears to be a rather parochial view of psychology.

THE MEETING OF EAST AND WEST

East and West come together in the melding of Eastern spiritual wisdom with Western scientific knowledge. The East has looked inside to discover the ultimate spiritual truths of existence. The West has looked outside to discover the powerful but relative truths of science. As psychology represents the West's scientific effort to understand the inner psyche, it becomes the common ground where these two great streams of knowing join, the natural meeting place of East and West.

To understand the depths of the human psyche, traditional psychology is necessary but not sufficient. Academic psychology and scientific psychology in the West have made a massive study of the outermost surface of the body, heart, and mind, and the depth psychologies fill out a deeper picture of our frontal organism. For the most part, Western psychology has now moved beyond the mind-body split that characterized much of psychological discourse during the first two-thirds of the 20th century to see this outer identity in holistic terms, that is, as an organismic, body-mind unity.

From an integral perspective, this is true as far as it goes. It does well represent our surface experience. But as we look farther, a more complex picture reveals itself. The self is only the outer edge of consciousness, where many inner strands of experience meet and fuse into a totality of organismic experiencing. But as Eastern psychology insists, a deeper, spiritual core manifests this outer mind, heart, and body. The frontal organism we identify with and call ourselves is an expression of our deeper being, and only in reference to this deeper foundation can there be a more complete psychological understanding.

Integral psychology begins with the ancient Vedantic conception of the *koshas*, or sheaths of consciousness. On the surface, these consist of the body, heart, and mind (*annamayakosha, pranayamayakosha, manomayakosha*) that form the human organism. Body, heart, and mind are precisely what Western psychology has studied. Indeed, this is *all* that is admitted by conventional psychology. But integral yoga charts three other levels of consciousness: the inner being, the true being, and the central being. These other three levels invisibly provide the foundation for this frontal organism we call our physical, emotional, mental self.

THE FRONTAL ORGANISM: THE MENTAL LEVEL

To understand the frontal body-heart-mind organism, we begin with the level of mind. Integral Vedanta charts three distinct parts of the mind, called the physical mind, the emotional mind, and the mind proper. This tripartite division has now been confirmed by recent developments in neuroscience. These three divisions correspond to what science now calls the triune brain: the reptilian brain stem that runs the body, the mammalian, emotional brain or limbic system, and humans' most recent evolutionary development, the neocortex, which is the seat of abstract thinking and language (Lewis, Amini, & Lannon, 2000).

While we share the lower, reptilian brain with lower animals, and we share the emotional brain or limbic system with mammals, allowing us to feel emotions and to experience an emotional connection to others, only human beings have a developed neocortex capable of abstract thought.

Medical research has generated much knowledge about the body and brain, and the examination of emotional and physical responses to our thinking patterns has led behaviorism and cognitive psychology to make some limited but significant contributions to psychotherapy, especially in the areas of depression and the continuum of stress, anxiety, fear, and panic. Cognitive therapy has shown how our thoughts (cognitions) significantly determine how we feel, and it also has proven effective for certain types of depression (Beck, 1979, 1985, 1987). Additionally, behaviorism's insights into the importance of relaxation in the treatment of stress, anxiety, panic, and phobias have had a major impact in this area of therapy. Behavior therapy is the treatment of choice for phobias and for certain kinds of symptom relief in anxiety and stress. But even though it can provide symptom relief for certain symptoms and even certain personality disorders, its power to bring about deeper change is limited, because it restricts its attempts to change to manipulating the surface components of conscious thinking and muscular tension.

Academic and behavioral approaches to psychology provide an explanation of the visible effects on the surface but not the deeper causes within. For this it is necessary to bring in the different schools of depth psychology. However, the many competing theories initially present a confusing picture. However, in seeing Western psychology within the organizing framework of integral psychology, it becomes clear that the various schools of psychology have each made a specialized study of particular levels of our being. *Different schools of psychology are windows into different levels of human consciousness.* Each major school of psychology is a vision of the whole seen through the level in which it specializes. From the vantage point of integral psychology, all of the conflicts and squabbling among the various schools of psychology are but conflicts between different levels of consciousness. Similarly, different Eastern systems tend to focus only on part of our inmost identity, and the conflicts between traditions stem from this difference in emphasis. Each school of psychology, Western or Eastern, is an important piece of the jigsaw puzzle.

The clinical branch of psychology has made understanding the dynamics of the psyche its field of study. As the depth psychologies have brought to light, *the center of the human psyche lies in the affective core of the self, our heart or emotional nature.*

THE EMOTIONAL LEVEL

What characterizes living beings is the vital principle, a vitality or life force (*prana*) that animates all living creatures. In human beings the vital principle manifests as the emotional level of the heart—our desires, our instincts, our feelings, our aspirations, our zest for living. Much of modern depth psychology can be read as rigorous research into the heart and emotions. Beginning with Freud's revolutionary discoveries about the unconscious, depth psychology has had an enormous impact upon the world and has shattered the view of the human being as the "rational animal" that had been humanity's self-image since Aristotle's time. As Freud plumbed the nonrational realms of the unconscious, a more modern account of psychological life emerged, in which desire, instinct, and strong emotional forces shape psychological life.

Depth psychology began over a century ago with Freud's search for ways to heal the sufferings of the human heart. In the process it uncovered the universal phenomenon of emotional wounding and how the human heart protects itself by developing defenses against this emotional wounding. In our family of origin there are failures to attune to the emotional state of the infant and young child, there are accidents, there are traumas, there is inevitable emotional pain growing up. The parents, who due to their own emotional wounding can only respond empathically to some of the child's emotions and self, tune out what is emotionally threatening. To cope with this and to maintain the vital bond with the parents, the child holds down this pain, represses certain impulses, and disavows certain feelings, and after a period of time, this all becomes automatic and unconscious. The child internalizes the parental prohibitions and develops a coping strategy that adapts to the family system, but in so doing adopts a false self that is alienated from the authentic self buried within. Large portions of the authentic self become unconscious and create deficits or gaps in the structure of the self, large areas of feeling and impulse become unconscious, the child dissociates from the body in the process, and so portions of physical awareness also fade away.

Integral yoga charts three gradations of the emotional level that range in frequency from greater density to greater refinement. At the lower end lies the lower emotional, our animal inheritance of primitive impulses and instincts. The central emotional level consists of the ordinary emotions and feelings that make up most of daily life. And the refinement of the higher emotional is the level most open to the creativity of our inner being, the light of spiritual experience, and our higher life aspirations.

While all schools of psychotherapy address the emotional level, psychoanalysis has charted this level most thoroughly. The three layers of the emotional correspond to the three major movements within psychoanalysis: classical psychoanalysis maps the lower emotional, contemporary psychoanalysis maps the central emotional, and Carl Jung's analytic psychology maps the higher emotional level.

The lower emotional is the realm of classical psychoanalysis that was popular during the first half of the 20th century. The lower emotional is the most animalistic part of our being, inherited from our long evolutionary past, called by Freud the "id." Freud's image of the id as "a seething cauldron of desire" vividly captures this dimension of the psyche. The lower emotional includes sexuality in all of its many libidinous forms, along with our aggressive impulses (Kahn, 2002).

Freud distilled two poles to our instinctual nature that he named Eros (sex) and Thanatos (aggression). The lower emotional encounters each experience through this lens of our biological urges and desire: "Can I eat it, mate with it, or kill it?" Sometimes we can be absorbed by the pure taste of food, its smells and textures. Other times we feel aggression and rage at the world and those who hurt us. Still other times we want to immerse ourselves in sexual passion, the instinctive yearning for the pleasures of erotic embrace.

This level translates all social interactions into its own terms. At this level we greet every new person with the inner questions: "Is this person friendly or hostile? Am I safe, or do I need to defend myself? Am I attracted to this person or not? Is this person a potential lover or a competitor?"

Freud began his psychoanalytic investigations toward the end of the Victorian era, a time when the repression of sexuality and the body was at its height in Western civilization. The lower emotional dimension looms large when it is strongly repressed, and naturally this is what emerged most forcefully when the lid of repression was lifted. Though Freud believed this level was the defining element of the psyche, in hindsight we can see that this exaggeration had an important evolutionary purpose—to bring to light our repressed animal nature as a universal dimension of human consciousness. Freud simply did what every major psychological theorist has done since—he took the discovery of one part of our being and viewed all the rest of the psyche through this lens.

Toward the end of his life, Freud shifted his focus from the id to the ego, which presaged the next significant shift in psychoanalytic thinking, namely, the emergence of object relations, self psychology, and intersubjectivity. What psychoanalysts such as Melanie Klein (1975a, 1975b), D. W. Winnicott (1967, 1971), W. R. D. Fairbairn (1954), and Heinz Kohut (1971, 1977, 1984) recognized, particularly as society itself changed and no longer was so repressive of the lower emotional, is that the self is more influenced by relationships than by instincts.

The central emotional level is the focus of study for Kohut's self psychology, the various schools of object relations, the interpersonal schools, family systems theories, the variety of intersubjective approaches, and all of what is generally referred to in contemporary psychoanalysis as the relational model. In the language of integral psychology, *it is not the lower emotional level that best characterizes the psychological world of most people but the central emotional level.*

The central emotional level sees the world through the sense of self and its relational world. The central emotional asks the questions: "Do I feel good, whole, with a healthy glow of self-esteem, or do I feel bad, fragmented, afraid of feeling ashamed or insufficient? Do others see me as effective and worthwhile, or as barely competent or faking it? Do I feel anxious, stressed, threatened in my interactions with others, or at ease, peaceful, secure? Are there people in my life who affirm and love me? Am I seen deeply for who I am? Are there others I respect, look up to, and feel reassured and strengthened by? Do I have loving, supportive, intimate relationships with close friends, partner, family, or am I estranged, afraid to share my true feelings, lonely, or not as intimately connected with others as I would like to be? Am I aligned with my deeper self's ambitions and actual talents, or do I feel alienated from work and career? Do I feel real and solid or somehow unreal, anxious, or vaguely uneasy? Do I have enough personal space and autonomy, or am I impinged upon, engulfed, my self subsumed by family and society?"

As most people today are centered in the central emotional level of their being, they are preoccupied by their sense of self and their relationships. Contemporary psychoanalysis sees the self as fundamentally relational and takes the central emotional as the defining dimension of human experience. *The self is the central organizing principle of the psyche, not the instincts.* This is the conceptual revolution within psychoanalysis that has occurred in the past several decades. However, from an integral perspective, it remains an incomplete description without reference to a third area, the higher emotional.

Carl Jung, one of Freud's two most gifted students, rebelled against the materialistic and reductionistic trends in Freud's thinking. Acknowledging the spiritual, the intuitive and creative, the validity of higher aspirations that cannot be reduced to thwarted sexual strivings or sublimated libido, Jung pioneered the mapping of the higher emotional level. The higher emotional is more open to the spiritual and operates at a more refined vibration than the lower or central emotional. Though it is not the source of our spiritual, artistic, philosophical, and higher strivings, the higher emotional is the most receptive to their influence.

In addition, the higher emotional takes on a mentalized quality. The higher emotional is the dreamer, the source of our plans and hopes, our visions of what can be, our strivings for beauty and for a better world. The higher emotional asks: "What is possible? What can I do, what can I create, what might I become? What leads toward a higher life?"

The higher emotional accesses the imaginal realm of visualization, imagination, and visionary experience. Being the part most open to the inner vital and its creative inspirations, it is no accident that Jung used active imagination and visualization as key therapeutic techniques in his therapy, for imagination is the coin of this realm.

Freud and classical psychoanalysis chart the lower emotional, contemporary psychoanalysis charts the central emotional level that typifies the average consciousness at this point in evolution, and Jung's analytic psychology charts the higher emotional realm. However, as the depth approaches of humanistic and existential psychology point out, this is still incomplete, because it fails to acknowledge the immense importance of the body.

THE PHYSICAL LEVEL

Our physical body is an extraordinary instrument, unique among all life-forms in its capacity to house the mind and consciousness of the human being. The Aitareya Upanishad relates a myth in which the gods (which in this symbolism represent the functions of the human mind) continued to reject one after another of the various animal bodies that the Divine Self offered to them. It was only when the human body was developed that the gods exclaimed, "This indeed is perfectly made," and consented to enter in.

Integral Vedanta's view that not only mind but our emotional life emerges out of the physical and retains its roots in bodily existence is shared and has been amplified by humanistic and existential schools of psychology. These depth approaches emphasize that *feeling life is embedded in bodily experience.* Wilhelm Reich, who along with Jung was the other of Freud's most gifted students, first recognized that emotional experience emerges from the body, and the humanistic and existential schools that followed developed this insight further.

Reich's theoretical heirs include Fritz Perls (1969; Perls, Hefferline, & Goodman, 1951) and gestalt therapy, Alexander Lowen (1975) and bioenergetics, Eugene Gendlin (1981, 1996) and focusing, John Pierrakos (1990) with core energetics, Ron Kurtz (1990) and hakomi, and the many other body-centered approaches, including Charlotte Selver's sensory awareness. Even Carl Rogers' (1961) client-centered therapy was theoretically grounded in the primacy of organismic experiencing. And while existential psychotherapy emerged from a different direction out of European philosophy (Yalom, 1980), its key concepts of actual lived experience and the importance of moving beyond intellect into bodily experiencing align closely with Reich's bodily focus. The explosion of body disciplines during the last decades of the 20th century led to a radical reevaluation of the importance of the body for full self-awareness.

The organism acts as an organized whole to create psychological experience. This is the conceptual revolution that humanistic-existential psychology has brought about, a holistic vision of psychological experience. Humanistic and existential schools confirm that childhood wounding not only brings about a lack of integration but also a dissociation of the self from the body that psychoanalysis overlooks. *Our defenses result in losing awareness of both our emotional and physical being.*

A complete vision of health must include not only integration and self-cohesion but also a more vibrant, sensorily alive state, a state with the joy, beauty, and pleasure that is the glory of embodiment.

At this level of bodily experience we ask, "Do I feel vibrantly alive, sensing and tasting what I do, from showering or walking, to sitting and talking? Or do I feel distracted from my sensory life, lost in my thoughts? Do I see the clouds and sky, or do I barely notice them? Do I experience my feelings as rooted in my body sensing, or am I hardly tuned in to them? Can I sense how my feelings live in me, energize me, course through my body? Am I aware of how verbalizing my feelings deepens my somatic experiencing of them? Do I feel how my breathing supports my excitement and the intensity of my feeling states, or do I find myself holding my breath, constricting my breathing and stifling my feelings? Do I feel grounded in my physical being or lost somewhere in my head?"

How rooted we are in bodily experiencing is difficult to assess, for everyone believes they are "in their body." In one sense everyone is right, because we are embodied beings. But there is a wide continuum of experiencing, ranging from a deep sense of being an embodied being-in-the-world to feeling like a mind "in" a body. Given how much dissociation is considered "normal" in our culture, there are very few people who have healed this split and are deeply rooted in their physical being.

No matter how cohesive the self may be, until the dissociation from the body is healed, the self will always feel some sense of unreality and vagueness. The physical dimension of self-experience gives concreteness to our experience, a quality of aliveness and sensory grounding that makes us realize in a definite way, "I exist now, here, grounded in this bodily form." For the body lives in the present, and when we come more fully into our body, we enter the domain of the eternal now, another area where humanistic and existential therapies converge.

THE LEVELS OF SELFHOOD

Organizing the various schools of psychology into the different levels of consciousness in which they specialize leads to the following simplified chart:

Mental level	**The Mental self**	Cognitive psychology
Higher emotional	**The Imaginal self**	Jungian psychology
Central emotional	**The Relational self**	Contemporary psycho-analysis, self psychology, object relations, intersubjectivity, family systems
Lower emotional	**The Instinctual self**	Classical psychoanalysis
Physical	**The Embodied self**	Humanistic and existential schools

Note that this chart is not a value hierarchy, for each level is important, but it is a hierarchy in density of consciousness. Each school of psychology has a unique gift to offer the world, a unique domain of consciousness that it illuminates. It must be emphasized that each school is not restricted to its chosen level. Just because the analytic traditions first charted the emotional level does not mean that the emotional is the exclusive province of psychoanalysis. *It is not that each school only addresses a particular part of our being, but that each school excels by its primary focus on one part, even as it downplays other parts of our being.*

It would be inaccurate, for example, to say that classical or contemporary psychoanalysis disregards the higher emotional or the body. On the contrary, psychoanalysis has made important contributions to the study of creativity and imagery. But psychoanalysis has concentrated its attention on the lower and central emotional, and the higher emotional, with its spiritual strivings, has been considerably deemphasized. Similarly, psychoanalysis does not completely ignore the body, but its map of consciousness so downplays this dimension of psychological experience that we need the discoveries of the somatic and existential therapies to adequately guide us here, while recognizing that they, too, tend to reduce everything to their level.

Due to that universal narcissistic tendency for each new discovery to be enthroned as the highest and best, each school annexes one part of our being, proclaims its centrality for human happiness, and stops there, translating the rest of our being through the lens of that level. The schools of psychology begin by liberating us, but, in the end, the particular level of consciousness in which each school specializes leads to a new cul-de-sac, a new limitation preventing further expansion. Unless there is a greater psychology that encompasses and goes beyond the conventional schools of psychology, there can be no release into the fullness of deeper being.

THE INNER REALMS OF BEING

This is where conventional psychology stops—a detailed and thorough mapping of our outer being—our body-heart-mind organism.

Only recently has psychology opened the door to the inner being through the transpersonal school. Perhaps now we are ready to admit the spiritual literature for what it is—rich phenomenological reports from thousands of individuals over many centuries. Eastern psychology provides important clinical data that can no longer be ignored or pathologized but must be accounted for by any psychology that tries to be inclusive. Transpersonal writers such as Stan Grof (1975, 1985, 1989), Ken Wilber (1986, 2000), Hameed Ali (Almaas, 1986, 1988, 1996), and Michael Washburn (1988, 1994) have provided provocative glimpses into the deeper realms of our inner being, although this territory has only been partially mapped.

In the West the first sense of something deeper was originally brought to light by Carl Jung. Jung made psychology's initial incursion into the inner being, and the archetypes of the collective unconscious immediately greet us in this domain. The collective unconscious serves as the psychological raw material out of which we construct our personal identity. In itself, it is a zone of transition between the cosmic forces and the human, where universal forces— universal emotional forces, physical forces, mental forces—take psychological shape. But the collective unconscious only exists by reference to what is beyond it, namely, the inner vital, inner mental, and subtle physical worlds.

Integral psychology delineates three inner realms of being that form the foundation for the frontal self: the *inner being*, the *true being*, and the *central being*. The first realm, the *inner being*, consists of an inner or subtle body, an inner heart or vital, and an inner mind. This layer of our inner being is a much enlarged, more powerful dimension of consciousness that is in direct touch with the universal forces of the intermediate plane. While wider, more fluid, and more expansive than our outer being, open to a larger scale and more subtle range of experience, the inner being is still of the same basic substance as the outer mind, heart, and body and therefore is more open to the cosmic forces of ignorance and darkness as well as to spiritual experiences. 2nd

The inner being opens to the intermediate plane, also sometimes called the astral plane, etheric plane, or subtle plane. This is a plane of experience that Eastern psychology has mapped extensively and is acknowledged by every spiritual tradition in the world. Native cultures and shamans view the world through this intermediate plane, and there is a considerable New Age fascination with the subtle energies and powers that can develop here, such as clairvoyance. Eastern traditions warn of the dangers here and advise the seeker not to get detoured by this sideshow, for the true goal lies beyond.

However important the intermediate plane is, it remains a very mixed realm of experience. But a beginning of definite spiritual experience can come by entering into the third realm, the true being. Here lies the true physical, true emotional, and true mental being (physical, emotional, mental *purusha*). This appears to be what Ali (A. H. Almaas) refers to as the world of "essence" and of Jung's "Self." The true being is a more essential spiritual plane, where the atman is represented on each of these levels, and it can be a point of entry into our impersonal spiritual nature.

The fourth, inmost level is the central being. What has not been clearly understood by the different Eastern traditions is the twofold nature of our spiritual identity, spirit and soul. Integral yoga elucidates how the central spiritual being is differentiated into the atman and the psychic being (or true soul). High above is the atman or Buddha-nature, the silent Self that is our universal identity with the Divine, eternal and nonevolving. Below, here within the manifestation, is our spiritual individuality, *antaratman* or psychic center, called in the Upanishads the *chaitya purusha*, our immortal, evolving soul. Atman and *antaratman* are the two aspects of our deepest spiritual nature that correspond to the Impersonal and Personal Divine, spirit and soul.

The atman can be experienced in its negative or *nirguna* aspect as Buddha-nature or pure emptiness, a vast space of nothingness, formless yet containing all form, without any qualities or attributes other than pure consciousness. This is the perspective of the Eastern psychologies of Buddhism, Taoism, *kevala advaita*, and certain tantric schools. In other schools of Vedanta, the atman also can be experienced in its positive or *saguna* aspect as the Self, a sea of consciousness, peace, light,

DUALITY

and knowledge that is spread out infinitely. Usually only experienced in Samadhi, there are overhead planes where this divine consciousness ascends into greater light, power, and knowledge, called by Sri Aurobindo higher mind, illumined mind, intuitive mind, overmind, and supermind.[1] Though the atman's native home is above in the overhead planes, it can descend into the manifestation and be experienced on any plane.

Enlightenment is the full realization of the atman or Self (and not just the temporary *experience* of atman). Enlightenment liberates a person from the ego, the separate sense of self. It is this realization that is known in Vedanta and Buddhism as nirvana, or extinction of the self. In place of the separate ego sense there remains the atman or Buddhanature.

The atman's identity is essentially one with the impersonal Brahman. It is this realization that is at the heart of *kevala advaita vedanta*. "Atman is Brahman, Brahman is atman," in the words of the Upanishads. The atman of one person is in essence the same as the atman of all others. Its characteristic is oneness, an identity of individual consciousness with Brahman. The metaphors of the river flowing into the sea or the drop of water dissolving into the ocean illustrate this loss of the lower individuality of ego in order to gain a higher identity with Brahman.

The atman stands outside the evolution, unaffected by the passing show of this ever-changing world. The realization of atman (or Buddha-nature) is the final goal of spiritual practice in *kevala advaita*, Buddhism and Taoism. Calm, unchanging spirit, the atman or Self is the detached, observing witness of this earthly manifestation, ever abiding in eternal peace and silence.

Integral Vedanta highlights not just the atman but the *antaratman* or soul. While integral psychology holds both aspects of the central being equally, initially there is greater emphasis upon the psychic center, because the soul's growth is the first order of business. Also, because the atman realization or enlightenment is so rare, at best perhaps one in several million, it is only an indirect influence on the lives of most seekers. It contributes a sense of peace and spaciousness, but until enlightenment occurs, it does not fundamentally alter the substance of the consciousness. The awakening of the true soul or psychic center, however, is far more accessible to the ordinary person, and it can become a palpable influence that fundamentally transforms our ordinary consciousness.

The word "soul" is the cause of much confusion in English. Historically in Europe over the last several hundred years, soul meant the self or ego, and even now it generally refers to our heart or to our heart and mind together. Soul can mean the deeper parts of the personality or even the capacity to feel intensely. Even when soul is used in its spiritual context of "the immortal soul" in Christianity, Islam, Hinduism, or Judaism, it implies an unchanging, eternal substance rather than a growing being, for traditional theistic religions have failed to understand the evolutionary dimension of the soul. To clarify this confusion of meanings, Sri Aurobindo coined the term "psychic being" or "psychic center" to refer to this eternal core of the human psyche, for "psyche" itself originally meant soul.

The psychic being or soul, *antaratman*, is described by the bhakti schools of Vedanta, as well as by the Western traditions of Christianity, Judaism, and Islam.[2] In integral yoga, the psychic center is the evolutionary element in human beings. Whereas our frontal self and organism are but temporary masks that we wear for this one brief lifetime, our psychic center is our deepest psychological core and most authentic self. As the psychic center slowly develops, its power to influence the frontal self or ego increases, and it begins to turn the person inward, toward the spiritual depths within.

> It is an ever-pure flame of the divinity in things and nothing that comes to it, nothing that enters into our experience can pollute its purity or extinguish the flame. This spiritual stuff is immaculate and luminous and, because it is perfectly luminous, it is immediately, intimately, directly aware of truth of being and truth of nature; it is deeply conscious of truth and good and beauty because truth and good and beauty are akin to its own native character, forms of something that is inherent in its own substance. It is aware also of all that contradicts these things, of all that deviates from its own native character, of falsehood and evil and the ugly and the unseemly; but it does not become these things nor is it touched or changed by these opposites of itself which so powerfully affect its outer instrumentation of mind, life and body. (Aurobindo, 1970, pp. 891–892)

QUOTE

CONTEMPLATING — MAGIC AWAKENS THIS

The awakening of the psychic being brings an immensity of relief from life's stresses, a source of deep peace and inner joy that ever bubbles forth like an eternal spring, an intrinsic loving presence that nourishes our inner life and the lives of those around us. It is the true pith of the self, what makes our self uniquely *ours*.

Different schools of psychology have been tentatively groping toward this inmost core but have not yet come upon it. Our deepest identity is our psychic center. Our frontal self and organism are an expression of this deeper source, and it must be placed at the very center of any comprehensive vision of psychology. According to integral psychology, as long as Western psychology fails to recognize the psychic center, it will miss the defining essence of the human being. This would be an ironic fate for a field whose entire purpose is to understand human nature.

INTEGRAL PSYCHOLOGY

Eastern psychology studies the inner dimensions of consciousness that are the foundation for the surface levels of the psyche (the frontal self) that Western psychology studies. The inner dimensions of consciousness can best be studied by the most sensitive instrument known to psychology—human consciousness. As more and more people have direct and personal experience with these inner realms of being, it becomes more difficult for psychology to ignore this domain of human experience.

The journey of plunging deep within to discover our true psychic center is hard to manage without some kind of psychological orientation, for so many of the barriers to this inner opening are psychological in nature. Without realizing it, depth psychology's various schools have charted the initial barriers to this inward deepening by bringing to light the heart's hurts and wounds, the unconscious defenses that compensate for this wounding, and the loss of awareness that results. When the schools of depth psychology are synthesized into an integral whole, then the full power of Western psychology's discoveries can be brought to bear on the greater work of awakening our real center.

In integral psychotherapy, every level of the self is healed, integrated, and allowed to unfold—physical, lower emotional, central emotional, higher emotional, mental. But this is not all, for the authentic

First
Find
Authentic Outer
Self → Then work
Eye (open → to grow psychic
chakra) center
Heart Inner Self
Psychic
Antaratman

Integrality   27

self, no matter how fully actualized and fulfilled, still operates in the darkness and obscurity of the superficial consciousness of this outward life. It needs a greater light by which to live, and this means awakening the psychic being (evolving soul) and bringing it forward. Integral authenticity means raising each level of our organism—body, heart, mind—to its highest level, guided and infused by the psychic center.

When all of these levels can be developed, our authentic nature comes forth. And as Eastern psychology reminds us, our *svabhava* (essential or authentic nature) can be a pathway to our inner, spiritual depths. The different Eastern traditions have generally emphasized only half of our core nature, either soul or atman (Buddha-nature), but integral psychology brings together both. Our central being is both personal and impersonal, becoming and being, dynamic and static.

All systems of depth psychology describe a frontal authentic self that is who we most truly are. Even though there is a profound depth dimension to this frontal self, Western psychology does not penetrate to its most inward spiritual core. Rather, Western psychological systems describe this authentic nature in entirely psychological terms—gestalt therapy calls it the wisdom of organismic self-regulation, existential therapies call it authenticity, self psychology uses the phrase nuclear self, object relations uses true self, Jung calls it the Self—but they are all pointing to a deeper, more authentic level of our being that is the key to a fulfilling life.

When we ignore this authentic self, we drift far from our true path and experience alienation, fragmentation, and psychological pain. On the other hand, when we follow our authentic self, we are led along a life path where relationships and career become ever more deeply satisfying and life becomes more coherent and integrated. The problem is that because of our childhood wounding we develop a false self that is cut off from our deeper essence. We do not know our authentic self or know only part of it. The many compromises we make in growing up lead us away from authentic living. The farther away we are from our authentic self, the more false our life becomes. Instead of coherence and integration, we have fragmentation and disorder. Most of our difficulties in life stem from this identification with our false self and inauthentic life.

While Western psychology studies the outer authentic self, Eastern psychology studies the inner roots of our essential nature. Different systems describe different facets of this inner being —soul, *antaratman, chaitya purusha*, spirit, atman, Buddha-nature. In integral psychology, the psychic center or evolving soul is our most essential individuality. The body-heart-mind is an expression of this deeper soul, an instrument or a vehicle through which our soul manifests in the world. When this psychic center is open, awake, guiding our way, life is a joyous spiritual adventure. When it is closed or covered over, life can be a nightmare of pain, frustration, and perplexity. Finding our center is the key to life's fulfillment.

It is the evolving soul in us, the psychic center that puts forth a new body-heart-mind each new lifetime and is behind the authentic self. As our journey opens into these inner realms of being, we come upon an inner source of peace, self-existent delight, radiant love, and tenderness that is the very fount of wholeness we are seeking. With sincere aspiration, our authentic, essential self can lead to this, for it has its origins in and is a surface expression of this evolutionary center within. Our true soul aspires always for "the good, the true, and the beautiful," as Plato so trenchantly put it, but only as this aspiration turns inward toward the spiritual life does it find its real goal.

Although Eastern and Western psychology both point to a deeper, authentic nature, they often travel in different, even opposite, directions to find it. For example, each of these two traditions relates to desire very differently. Western psychology charts the unfolding of desire as the path to fulfillment. Eastern psychology, on the other hand, speaks of the refinement and transcendence of desire as the path to fulfillment. At first glance these seem to be mutually exclusive paths, but there is a larger unity to which these different traditions are pointing, a hidden harmony in which their seeming divergences converge and their contradictions are reconciled.

In today's world, with access to the riches of the world's psychological traditions, an integral vision of psychology can at last be formulated. Western psychology lacks an integrating framework and meaningful context by which to understand its extraordinary discoveries. Eastern psychology lacks a way to overcome the dense unconsciousness of the self's defensive structures, which pull ever downward. Only by enlarging psychology to include the inmost depths can we construct a true psychology of wholeness. This is the meeting of East and West, a union of the West's outer, empirical science of psychology with the East's inner, spiritual science of consciousness.

Chapter 2

Our Psychic Center

The pure psychic being is of the essence of Ananda, it comes from the delight-soul in the universe; but the superficial heart of emotion is overborne by the conflicting appearances of the world and suffers many reactions of grief, fear, depression, passion, shortlived and partial joy.
—Sri Aurobindo, *Synthesis of Yoga*

The finding of our true psychic center and the practical means for unveiling it are perhaps the most significant contributions of integral psychology to human welfare, for the discovery of our psychic center profoundly changes the entire experience of living. Instead of the stressful play of opposites that characterizes normal living—pleasure and pain, frustration and satisfaction, hope and despair—there is a steady light of inner guidance, a peaceful, loving presence that is ever fresh, ever new, a joyous, self-existent bliss in the center of our being.

It is an extraordinary notion that the essence of our deepest identity is a self-existent joy, an immense peace, an unfaltering guidance and discernment, an inexpressible sweetness, love, and light. This view runs so counter to prevailing psychological thought as to be revolutionary. Yet this is precisely what Eastern psychology has confirmed for thousands of years. Integral psychology reorients psychology from its exclusive preoccupation with the frontal self and organism to include the deeper, guiding psychic center within.

29

The Central Being

As discussed earlier, our fundamental identity is spiritual, and this central spiritual identity consists of two aspects, called by various names: spirit, atman, Self, Buddha-nature, on the one hand, and soul, psychic center, psychic being, *antaratman, chaitya purusha,* on the other. The Self or atman is our eternal, unevolving oneness with Brahman, the Divine. It stands outside the evolution—silent, detached, impartial, and unaffected by life. The soul or psychic center, however, participates in the evolution and itself undergoes a dynamic development. It is both immortal and growing in the evolution, developing new powers and capacities in each lifetime, actualizing new potentials in its journey toward maturity.

Bringing the outer body to God

The ancient, effulgent being, the indwelling spirit, subtle, deep-hidden in the lotus of the Heart, is hard to know. But the wise person following the path of meditation, knows him and is freed alike from pleasures and pain. (*Katha Upanishad*, pp. 17–18)

The Upanishads are generally regarded as the high point of Vedantic philosophy, and in the Upanishads it is the *chaitya purusha,* located in the secret cave in the heart, that corresponds to the psychic center.

According to the ancient teaching the seat of the immanent Divine, the hidden Purusha, is in the mystic heart—the secret heart-cave, *hrdaye guhâyâm,* as the Upanishads put it—and, according to the experience of many Yogins, it is from its depths that there comes the voice or the breath of the inner oracle. (Aurobindo, 1973b, p. 149)

It must be remembered that the psychic center is not located in the physical heart or in the heart *chakra,* though it is often confused with this heart center. It is located behind the heart chakra, deep within on an inner plane. The many images of the Christ pointing to his own open heart confirm Christ as the great Western teacher of this inmost soul within the heart, for the opening of the heart chakra is a precondition for the full emergence of the psychic center.

The psychic being in the old systems was spoken of as the Purusha in the heart (the secret heart—*hrdaye guhayam*) which corresponds very well to what we define as the psychic being behind the heart centre. It was also this that went out from the body at death and persisted—which again corresponds to our teaching that it is this which goes out and returns, linking a new life to former life. Also we say that the psychic is the divine portion within us—so too the Purusha in the heart is described as Ishwara [Personal Divine] of the individual nature. (Aurobindo, 1971a, p. 289)

All theistic traditions focus on the centrality of the soul—Christianity, Judaism, Islam, bhakti schools of Vedanta. All theistic traditions view our inmost identity as an immortal soul. What integral yoga adds to these descriptions is the evolutionary aspect of the soul. Sri Aurobindo's writing is unparalleled in its rich phenomenological descriptions of the actual experience of the soul or psychic center. The significance of the soul as our evolutionary guide could not have been appreciated by the earlier theistic traditions, because the evolutionary nature of the cosmos was not yet emphasized. The significance of the psychic center as the evolutionary principle within us becomes clear only as the evolution of consciousness is seen as the great theme of world existence. However, even as far back as the Vedas there was an awareness of the soul's upward movement and of the importance of the soul's guidance in this process.

The evolutionary nature of the soul can be confusing, for it is both an eternal and indestructible portion of the Divine and simultaneously a growing, developing center of consciousness. It is initially a seed of potential that contains all Divine possibilities within it. Its growth is a process of unfolding these latent powers. The psychic center is spirit in manifestation, ever alive, ever whole, ever pure, yet also progressing as it evolves new abilities out of itself. We are accustomed to think that eternal = static or pure being, but this applies only to the atman, the immobile, nonevolving portion of our spiritual nature. Eternal also can be in the mode of becoming, and it is this becoming that completes our spiritual identity and fulfills the evolutionary movement of the Divine creation. We are both an eternal *being* and *becoming*, at one level a static, silent witness that supports all impartially while simultaneously, on

aother level, an evolving becoming, a divine participant on the world
stage growing toward fullness.

> It is necessary to understand clearly the difference between the
> evolving soul (psychic being) and the pure Atman, self or spirit.
> The pure self is unborn, does not pass through death or birth,
> is independent of birth or body, mind or life or this manifested
> Nature. It is not bound by these things, not limited, not
> affected, even though it assumes and supports them. The soul,
> on the contrary, is something that comes down into birth and
> passes through death—although it itself does not die, for it is
> immortal—from one state to another, from the earth plane to
> other planes and back again to the earth-existence. It goes on
> with this progression from life to life through an evolution
> which leads it up to the human state and evolves through it all
> a being of itself which we call the psychic being that supports
> the evolution and develops a physical, a vital, a mental human
> consciousness as its instruments of world-experience and of a
> disguised, imperfect, but growing self-expression. All this it
> does from behind a veil showing something of its divine self
> only insofar as the imperfection of the instrumental being will
> allow it. But a time comes when it is able to prepare to come
> out from behind the veil, to take command and turn all the
> instrumental nature towards a divine fulfillment. This is the
> beginning of the true spiritual life. The soul is now able to
> make itself ready for a higher evolution of manifested con-
> sciousness than the mental human—it can pass from the
> mental to the spiritual and through degrees of the spiritual to
> the supramental state. Till then there is no reason why it should
> cease from birth, it cannot in fact do so. If having reached the
> spiritual state, it wills to pass out of the terrestrial manifesta-
> tion, it may indeed do so—but there is also possible a higher
> manifestation, in the Knowledge and not in the Ignorance.
> (Aurobindo, 1971a, pp. 438–439)

In the spiritual history of humanity it appears that full enlightenment, or the permanent realization of atman or Buddha-nature, is
exceedingly rare. There are probably no more than a handful of fully

enlightened beings on earth at a given time. However, consciousness of the psychic center is a far more available and common experience, and its realization leads not away from the earth plane but to an active involvement with earth's ongoing evolution. As the aforementioned quote implies, the psychic emergence is the flowering of the evolutionary journey and the beginning of another step in humanity's evolutionary progress. Such a transformation requires a continuity in identity, and this means the realization of the soul, our true spiritual individuality.

Integral yoga psychology begins with the assumption that this universe does have a purpose, so that simply to nullify existence through nirvanic extinction cannot be the entire meaning of life. In seeing our life's journey as an evolution of consciousness, discovering our psychic center assumes the highest importance, since it is through our true identity that we can more consciously and creatively participate in the miracle of this living universe. The increasing influence of the psychic center is not only accessible to ordinary people, it also is the path of fulfillment in daily living, for it holds the key to finding our way amidst the confusion of the world around us.

THE NATURE AND GROWTH
OF OUR PSYCHIC CENTER

The experience of the psychic center is of a self-existent bliss, an intense inner happiness. A very palpable sense of joy is usually the first thing that greets us as the psychic center awakens. This strong joy is in no way dependent upon outer circumstances. It is intrinsic to the psychic being. Its essential nature is ever possessed of an exquisite, indescribable contentment and utter fulfillment.

This is a fulfillment that is unlike any other, for it is a fulfillment that does not simply bask in itself or remain static. This is a dynamic fulfillment that is energizing, inspiring, and seeks creative expression and further divine fulfillment. The experience of this inherent joy far surpasses the fleeting, surface satisfactions of regular life. Although people seek satisfaction through people and things, religious traditions suggest that it is this inner, spiritual wholeness that is being sought through these outer pursuits. A single taste of this psychic happiness can be enough to change the direction of a person's life, for it opens us to possibilities undreamed of before. For many people it is just such an experience that marks the beginning of the spiritual journey.

Along with this unparalleled contentment comes an inner quietude and a deep peace, in the biblical phrase, "the peace that passeth all understanding." This peace comes from deep within, and when it extends to the surface it brings a tranquility and calm to the mind and heart. This sense of peace brings an overpowering relief from the stress and anxiety that so pervade everyday life. It brings a comfort and solace that relieve our cares and burdens.

Spiritual traditions also concur that to experience soul is to experience a vastness of love and compassion that makes the ordinary experience of these feelings pale in comparison. Jesus Christ is the best known exemplar in the West of the realization of the soul and the possibilities that can manifest with the psychic transformation. Christ emphasized the power of love in the experience of the soul, and it is no accident that all theistic traditions have a strong orientation toward the heart, along with practices of love and devotion. In experiencing the vastness of spiritual love, we see what a diminished figure love assumes in everyday life, even as it originates from this deeper, purer immensity. The psychic center feels a loving kinship with all other beings and the whole of creation. And most of all, the psychic center feels a loving relationship with the Divine, for it brings an awareness of the Presence of the Divine. As a portion of the Divine, it aspires for full union. As the experience of the psychic center grows, the awareness of the Divine grows stronger and more clear and definite.

The psychic center moves always toward harmony, truth, beauty, goodness, and tenderness. Its intrinsic nature is spiritual, and to these higher spiritual values it is irresistibly attracted. But at first its voice is overshadowed by the clamor of the body, heart, and mind.

Every living being has a spark of the Divine within. This spark soul is present in every bacteria and unicellular organism. The atman at this beginning evolutionary stage is identical to the atman at all other evolutionary stages, but the psychic center, though its potential is fully present, has yet to be unfolded and actualized. In plants this psychic presence becomes stronger and more developed, but it remains a spark. In animals this psychic presence becomes stronger and better defined, as anyone sensitive to animals can feel. There is a beginning of mind in animals and therefore a greater means of expression than in plants, but in animals this mentality is still barely developed and is imprisoned by the senses.

Psychic development reaches a new stage in human beings. Here the spark has become a flame. A definite psychic center has been formed, though it is still far from maturity. In the first stages of human evolution, this psychic center continues to focus on building up the body, heart, and mind and has little influence on the life of the person. Developing the frontal, instrumental nature is its first task, as the outwardness and density of the surface instruments obscure the soul's inner intimations. During these first stages of the human level, the person is almost completely lost in the outer world, seeking only to satisfy physical, emotional, and mental desires. The surface instruments run the whole show.

As the psychic center progresses it works to refine and purify this frontal nature so that body, heart, and mind will be responsive to this light and take their true place as instruments that express the inner soul. The guidance of the psychic center is a direct form of spiritual knowing, for the psychic has within it a discernment that is not misled by outer appearances but can see beyond to the deeper truth that surface appearances often hide.[1] In our life journey, our psychic center is our true guide.

As the psychic center matures and grows stronger, it exerts an increasing influence upon the frontal nature, and the person begins to turn inward, to experience a greater depth in living rather than being confined to the superficial life of the surface. Our psychic center draws us toward higher, more noble things in life. It is what attracts us to genuine love, to truth, to beauty, to peace, to bliss, to people whose hearts are open and whom we feel nourished by, to real tenderness, to shining joy and exuberance, to honest, truthful people, to those who strive for a higher way of life, to authenticity, to health, to wholeness. Sometimes, especially when the psychic center is less developed, we are attracted to an image of these things and get lost in the outer appearances, such as sentimental piety, proclamations of love but not its inner feeling, raucous energy, blind passion, moralistic rules, or even repressive Puritanism. But such mistakes are necessary in the soul's growth, for by trial and error we learn the difference between surface appearances, desires, and our deeper psychic guidance.

Through this the psychic center becomes stronger, more insistent, more able to influence the frontal self. It acts to edify and cleanse our frontal nature so that we can choose more freely and clearly, less enslaved by the insistence of our impulses and emotional nature. As the psychic center awakens, it brings a guidance, a light, a new and deeper perspective that changes the orientation of the person and leads him or her inward.

> There are always two different consciousnesses in the human being, one outward in which he ordinarily lives, the other inward and concealed of which he knows nothing. When one does sadhana, the inner consciousness begins to open and one is able to go inside and have all kinds of experiences there. As the sadhana progresses, one begins to live more and more in this inner being and the outer becomes more and more superficial. At first the inner consciousness seems to be the dream and the outer the waking reality. Afterwards the inner consciousness becomes the reality and the outer is felt by many as a dream or delusion, or else as something superficial and external. The inner consciousness begins to be a place of deep peace, light, happiness, love, closeness to the Divine or the presence of the Divine, the Mother. One is then aware of two consciousnesses, the inner one and the outer which has to be changed into its counterpart and instrument. (Aurobindo, 1971a, p. 307)

At first these are two seemingly unrelated worlds—the inner spiritual world and the outer world of regular life. Though the inner light seems faint at first, gradually it becomes brighter. Over time, this light shines farther outward and begins to illumine our way in the outer world, even as it is still easily overshadowed by our mental patterns and emotional preferences and habits. Indeed, as we shall see, it is our wounding, our unconscious defenses, and our emotional reactivity that are the greatest barriers to the psychic light. To fully liberate this light is a goal of integral psychology.

This process of psychic emergence, of living in two parallel worlds or consciousnesses, is difficult to navigate at times. It is easy to doubt or dismiss what is occurring when the inner world is just starting to open, because it is so easily overcome by the momentum of the frontal self. For a long time, these two worlds may seem very distinct and separate, like oil and water. But through sustained practice and aspiration, the psychic light grows stronger. Progressively, it becomes a guiding force in daily life, not separate from but part of outer living. Finally, as the psychic influence pervades the body, heart, and mind and transforms these surface instruments, at last the psychic center comes to the front of the consciousness and takes direct charge of the organism, opening the person fully to the spiritual realm.

As the crust of the outer nature cracks, as the walls of inner separation break down, the inner light gets through, the inner fire burns in the heart, the substance of the nature and the stuff of consciousness refine to a greater subtlety and purity, and the deeper psychic experiences, those which are not solely of an inner mental or inner vital character, become possible in this subtler, purer, finer substance; the soul begins to unveil itself, the psychic personality reaches its full stature. The soul, the psychic entity, then manifests itself as the central being which upholds mind and life and body and supports all the other powers and functions of the Spirit; it takes up its greater function as the guide and ruler of the nature. A guidance, a governance begins from within which exposes every movement to the light of Truth, repels what is false, obscure, opposed to the divine realization: every region of the being, every nook and corner of it . . . is lighted up with the unerring psychic light, their confusions dissipated, their tangles disentangled, their self-deceptions precisely indicated and removed; all is purified, set right, the whole nature harmonized, modulated in the psychic key, put in spiritual order. This process may be rapid or tardy according to the amount of obscurity and resistance still left in the nature, but it goes on unfalteringly so long as it is not complete.

This is the first result, but the second is a free inflow of all kinds of spiritual experience, experience of the Self, experience of the Ishwara and the Divine Shakti, experience of cosmic consciousness, a direct touch with cosmic forces and with the occult movements of universal Nature, a psychic sympathy and unity and inner communication and interchanges of all kinds with other beings and with Nature, illuminations of the mind by knowledge, illuminations of the heart by love and devotion and spiritual joy and ecstasy, illuminations of the sense and the body by higher experience, illuminations of dynamic action in the truth and largeness of a purified mind and heart and soul, the certitudes of the divine light and guidance, the joy and power of the divine force working in the will and the conduct. These experiences are the result of an opening outward of the inner and inmost being and nature; for then there comes into play the soul's power of unerring inherent consciousness, its vision, its touch on things which is superior to any mental cognition; there is there, native to the psychic consciousness in its pure working, an immediate sense of the world and its beings, a direct inner contact with them and a direct contact with the Self and with the Divine—a direct knowledge, a direct sight of Truth and of all truths, a direct penetrating spiritual emotion and feeling, a direct intuition of right will and right action, a power to rule and to create an order of the being not by the gropings of the superficial self, but from within, from the inner truth of self and things. (Aurobindo, 1970, pp. 907–908)

The psychic transformation occurs by degrees. First there is an opening to our psychic center, an experience that profoundly reorients our life and direction. Difficulties, pain, trials, and suffering still come as they do to everyone, but there is a center of bliss inside that no outer event can touch. Mistakes are still made, since we cannot listen perfectly to the deeper guidance, and the surface self's habitual reactions have a strong forward thrust. But slowly, as the psychic center awakens, it becomes a guiding force in our lives. This inner guidance also protects us from the dangers of the inner journey, for in integral yoga psychology the psychic center brings discernment (*viveka*) and is the only part of the being that cannot be touched by the tempting powers of the intermediate zone. As this proceeds our life harmonizes with our inner being, so that all parts of our existence become increasingly aligned with our deeper psychic center—our work, our play, our relationships, our diet, our exercise, our entertainment, the books we read, the influences and experiences to which we are open. In this process the ego becomes more and more transparent, purified, receptive to the psychic's direction. The frontal self undergoes a psychic transformation that thoroughly alters its makeup.

In Western psychology, however, our psychic center is viewed from the perspective of our ordinary, frontal self. To more clearly understand the psychic center or true soul, it is necessary to consider what it is confused with by Western psychology and hides it—the ego, the self.

WESTERN UNDERSTANDINGS OF OUR PSYCHIC CENTER

We all experience life from the perspective of a subjective self, an ego, the sense of "I." It is a fact of our daily life. What is the essence of this "I"-ness? It lies in this: the feeling of identity, of being a person, a subjectivity. It is not only a sense of presence or being or existence but of being *a* presence, *a* being, *an* existence, the experience and feeling of, "I am, I exist." From where does this fundamental source of selfhood come? What exactly is this self we so take for granted? Why do we have a self or, rather, why are we a self? Further, amidst all this continual flux and flow, why is it that we experience our self as being continuous and stable? Is this merely an illusion? Or is there a deeper reality to our psyche that radiates out to our surface experience? Is what we take to be our self actually our real identity? What lies at the core of our being?

What Western psychology has studied in great detail is the self, the ego. In conventional psychology, the ego is generally regarded as the center of psychological life. Psychoanalytic theory even goes so far as to define the ego as "the seat of consciousness." Further, it delineates numerous characteristics and functions of the ego, such as reality testing, memory, the control of motility and impulse control, orientation in space, and it is the center of perception. It integrates the demands of external reality with inner psychological life, resulting in the development of the unconscious, for the ego controls the unconscious defense mechanisms that keep unacceptable feelings and parts of the self out of awareness.

Yet despite how much psychology has learned about the self, there remain fundamental questions that cannot be resolved within the paradigm of conventional psychology, for Western psychology, like all of science, starts from the surface appearance of things and tries to understand the deeper structure from without. But this method has definite limits in the field of psychology. Traditional psychology has been unable to plumb the inner depths of the psyche, because its methodology of empirical observation can only go as far as the physical mind can go. It is unable to see beyond into our deeper being. The self, for all that psychology has learned about it, remains a mystery.

CURRENT VIEWS OF THE SELF

Beginning with Freud's investigations into "das Ich" (the "I"), the self has been the central focus of inquiry for the field of psychology. James Strachey, the original German translator of Freud, tried to impress upon his English-speaking audience the scientific nature of Freud's work and so translated "das Ich" into the Latin term *ego*. Although Freud used ego in two different ways, as self and as mental apparatus, usage in most psychoanalytic circles today has developed to where ego and self are used interchangeably.

The most sophisticated understanding of the self comes from the current object relations and self psychology schools of psychoanalysis, which have made a detailed study of the origins and structure of the self (Fairbairn, 1954; Guntrip, 1969; Jacobson, 1964; Kernberg, 1975, 1980; Klein, 1975a, 1975b; Winnicott, 1958, 1965, 1971; Kohut, 1971, 1977, 1984). Object relations theory describes the self as a growing composite of images that begins to take shape from the moment of birth. From its earliest experiences, the infant begins to take raw bits of undifferentiated experience and organizes these into emotionally charged images of self and other (or "objects"). The first distinction is between inside and outside, me and not me (Klein, 1975b). Then the various images, good and bad, helpful and hurtful, consolidate to form stable images of self and others. Based on our earliest relationships, especially with our mother and father, we internalize images of ourselves and others, slowly building up internal representations of the self and other. The infant's capacity for perception and memory and for establishing representations of itself and others is furthered by the development of symbolic and abstract thinking. We construct an internal world with an integrated sense of self and an integrated sense of others, a "representational world," a kind of virtual reality that becomes for us our experience of ourselves and the world. It organizes an otherwise chaotic internal and external experience.

This process continues through our entire life cycle. We continually add to and take away from this self system as our life unfolds, just as we continually modify our image system of the world. However, although the self and object world are under continual construction and modification, the more superficial layers of this image usually undergo change, as much of our enduring sense of self is established by age six or seven. The self is powerfully molded by our earliest experiences in our family of origin and lays down the foundational images of self and other in these early years. *The emotional wounding we all experience in childhood is instrumental in forming this early representational world.* One aftermath of this early wounding is the development of the unconscious where forbidden feelings and impulses are relegated, a defensive system for keeping portions of the self off-limits, and the arrest of major developmental lines of the self, which results in deficits in the structure of the self.

When certain developmental needs are unmet or traumatized, in effect this freezes the developmental process in significant areas of the self. And as behaviorism has shown, the first time we are exposed to a new situation, especially a situation that has a high degree of arousal and emotional intensity, this learning has a particular power for forming long-lasting impressions. This is known as "the primacy effect" and forms a kind of template or lens that shapes how we view similar experiences in the future. The self adapts to the conditions of the original family system so that it can best maintain its vital ties with mother, father, and other caregivers. The primacy effect of childhood experiences in our family creates a profound and lasting imprint upon our psychic structure and self-image. Neurologically, these early experiences create neural networks that are strengthened over time and tend to override alternative pathways, becoming fixed grooves that reinforce these same neural circuits and allow new pathways to develop only under special conditions.

These imprints and neural pathways, in fact, are so strong that they are modified only under certain conditions, conditions rarely found outside of the special situation of intensive psychotherapy. They cannot be deeply modified merely by cognitive techniques, for this only affects the surface self and leaves the more deeply held structures of the self untouched. Real fundamental change to the self structure needs to be a deeply emotional experience, just as the original conditioning occurred in a deeply charged atmosphere of intense affects. Only a concentrated, contained environment such as is found in depth psychotherapy can replicate the original conditions in order to remobilize the derailed developmental needs so that deep and lasting change can occur.

This view of the self is very appealing and has a good deal of explanatory value. It explains why people behave emotionally and relate to others, particularly their most intimate relationships, along the lines of childhood patterns, even though they may function well in a given role or professional career. It explains why people get into marriages and friendships that tend to repeat ongoing dysfunctional patterns. It explains a great deal of neurosis and human unhappiness, and it even shows ways to heal and restore development.

However, there are other things it does not explain.

- It does not explain why we experience ourselves as a self, a person, for in this view the self is a kind of empty shell or holographic image with nothing within it. The self becomes a new version of the "ghost in the machine." It explains the self-image but not the self. *WHO'S DOING THE OBSERVING?*
- It does not explain why the self is experienced as a stable continuity.
- It does not explain the higher motivations of the self or its spiritual aspirations. *don't Actually it pretends they Exist — Ellie*

To deal with some of these problems many people have turned to Buddhism for an explanation, for object relations theory fits in nicely with the Eastern psychological views of Buddhism that see the self as a series of self-images that is fundamentally empty. Buddhist psychology has performed an even more microscopic examination of the self than object relations and has emerged with a more thorough deconstruction of the self. Buddhist texts report that when the self becomes the object of meditative inquiry, in looking closely at the images of the self it is discovered that there are spaces between these images. There actually is nothing to hold these images together. In meditatively penetrating the spaces between the images, it is found that there is no self, and emptiness is seen to be fundamental. It is this deeply experienced insight that liberates the person and leads to enlightenment.

The continuity of the self is explained as a kind of optical illusion, similar to watching movement in a movie. Although in watching a movie we see continuous movement, in reality we are looking at a series of rapidly flickering still photos that we interpret as continuous motion. The illusion of the continuity of the self is based upon a similar misperception. Thus Buddhist and object relations views of the self as an image converge, and the conclusion that the self is an illusion can seem convincing. Further, the Buddhists argue (along with the *kevala advaita Vedantins*) that if the self is not an illusion, then how can it drop away in enlightenment and never return, as the spiritual literature clearly documents? If the ego really is real, then how can it disappear? It disappears because it never was real to begin with, goes the argument.

However, there are several problems with this position. First, the explanation of the self as *only* an image or a composite of images is incomplete. Why should a self-image give rise to the feeling of being a being or "I"-ness? Why does the self-image not remain an empty series of images, for images lead only to more images, not to a palpable sense of inner being or personhood. From self-image to self is a gigantic leap that object relations and Buddhist descriptions fall short of explaining. Indeed, from Buddhism we get the statement that the self *is* empty, devoid of a true being or soul. But from where does our feeling of identity come? Why do we sense ourselves as *a being,* as a person?

This description of self as self-image explains neither the intrinsic sense of selfhood nor the continuity of the self. The metaphor of the movie projector to clarify the continuity of the self rests on static images of the self with gaps between these static images. But are there any such static images at all? Upon closer inspection we find that these apparently static images are not at all static but are put together moment to moment. The self-image is really *a self-imaging process* that is being constructed in each moment. There are no static images anywhere, not in the actual imaging process itself or in the spaces between. There is *only* movement and flow.

So from where does the sense of continuity come, for from discontinuity and flux we get only further discontinuity and flux, not continuity and stability. To dismiss continuity as only an illusion is to explain away the problem rather than provide genuine understanding. The ego's sense of identity and feeling of selfhood cannot be understood at the level of the self-image. The self-image is a surface reflection of a deeper reality, and attempting to analyze this is like attempting to dissect a mirage or holographic image. Of course, it appears empty and without inherent substance, just as Buddhist texts insist. But this is only its husk or outer form, not its central reality or inner essence. An analysis that restricts itself to the self's frontal appearance, no matter how thorough and microscopic this analysis may be, will fall short of a comprehensive understanding. It is only by reference to something beyond the self that the self can be understood more fully.

SVABHAVA

From an integral perspective, both the sense of self and the sense of continuity emanate from our psychic center, our true soul. Without reference to this eternal soul the experience of selfhood cannot be understood. Object relations and Buddhism are committed to worldviews that exclude the soul and are therefore unable to grasp central aspects of the experience of self. Here we find that psychoanalytic self psychology provides some help.

Self psychology accepts the reality of the self more fully than object relations or intersubjective approaches that see only self-other images. Kohut defines the self as "an independent center of initiative that is continuous in time and space" (Kohut, 1971). While contemporary trends in self psychology focus more on self experience than on metapsychological theory, traditional self psychology fleshes out three lines of development as being especially important. There is a line of expansive ambitions, an area of skills and talents, and a line of ideals and idealization (Kohut, 1971, 1977, 1984.) This recasts the psychological content of Freud's tripartite id-ego-superego while discarding the clumsy mental apparatus model of the mind that became so theoretically problematic for conventional psychoanalysis (and both Freud's and Kohut's models can be seen as a way of describing the lower emotional, central emotional, and higher emotional levels of the heart). But from where does this "center of initiative" come?

Self psychology reaches to what Kohut called the "nuclear self," a seed of potential from which the self emerges. Unfortunately, this concept is limited by Kohut's tether to his roots in classical psychoanalysis in its attribution of the origins of this seed to the earliest relationship with the mother and father. The "nuclear self" contains the "nuclear program" for the self, the capacities and direction for life that require sustaining, supporting human relationships in order to unfold throughout the life cycle. Self psychology is not alone in looking beyond the self for the source of the self. Most depth systems use some version of this explanation. In gestalt therapy, the self emerges from the organism, and as Perls (1969) said, "The ego knows very little, the organism knows everything." Existential therapy speaks of the "authentic self" that emerges from the ground of being. Jungian psychology refers to the archetype of the Self as the organizing principle for the ego. All of these are powerful speculations that seem to point to something similar, namely, a source beyond the ego of identity and potential, some greater ground of wisdom from which the self emerges.

These theories begin to touch upon the outer half of a more precise Vedantic conception of *svabhava*, defined earlier as intrinsic nature, essential self, or natural constitution. Vedantic psychology holds that our true psychic center is the soul, called the *chaitya purusha* or *antaratman* in the Upanishads, and is the real spiritual person within, our evolving soul. Each unique "soul is a force of self-consciousness that formulates an idea of the Divine in it and guides by that its action and evolution, its progressive self-finding, its constantly varying self-expression. . . . That is our Svabhava, our own real nature" (Aurobindo, 1973b, p. 502).

In this material world, however, the psychic center expresses itself by putting forward a unique body-heart-mind complex that, in the early stages of evolution, is barely or poorly attuned to its deeper nature.

> There too it acts, but is not in full possession of itself, is seeking as it were for its own true law in a half-light or a darkness and goes on its way through many lower forms, many false forms, endless imperfections, perversions, self-losings, self-findings, seekings after norm and rule before it arrives at self-discovery. . . . It is always Svabhava that is looking for self-expression and self-finding through all these things, a truth which should teach us universal charity and equality of vision, since we are all subject to the same perplexity and struggle. These motions belong, not to the soul, but to the nature. (Aurobindo, 1972a, p. 503)

Western psychology has made an extensive study of this frontal organism and self, and this frontal self is seen to emerge from a deeper "nuclear self" (or organism or authentic nature). This idea is remarkably similar to the *svabhava* or essential self that integral Vedanta describes. In integral psychology, the origins of the self lie not with the parents, as traditional psychoanalysis suggests, but rather in the essential self with which we are born. As any discerning parent can see, each new child comes into this world with a highly differentiated, unique essence that goes far beyond what each parent contributes genetically or historically, even though this essential nature is profoundly shaped by early experience. In integral psychology, neither the ego nor the authentic self can be adequately comprehended without reference to the psychic center.

It is from our psychic center that our sense of self ultimately derives. The psychic center manifests this instrumental nature and infuses our organismic existence with its sense of identity, and the various self-images and identifications form its outward skeletal structure. The psychic center fills in this skeletal structure of the self-image to provide the feeling of being a person, a being. It is because of the deeper soul that we have the phenomenological experience of being an existence, a presence, instead of being an empty succession of images with no person within. Integral psychology suggests that the self's sense of stability and continuity is present because it reflects a deeper spiritual fact of our existence, the eternity of our soul. Continuity and stability are facts of our deepest, most essential being and reflected on our surface experience, animate, and fill out the self-image to produce the feeling of stable, continuous selfhood.

Conventional psychology looks to the body, heart, and mind to explain our sense of selfhood and aliveness, but this fundamental sense of being transcends and is not reducible to physical sensations, emotions, or mental images. It resides deeper in our spiritual center. Our uniqueness and most essential identity is our soul, our true individuality, and all theories of the self that omit this will be lacking. A more comprehensive psychology is necessary, one that is not afraid of all things spiritual lest it appear unscientific, for if spirit is the fundamental nature of reality, then both reason and science demand that we pursue this wherever it may lead us.

If, as the highest wisdom of Eastern (and Western) cultures has affirmed for millennia, our psychic center is an eternal spiritual being, if our frontal organism is only a temporary vesture worn by our deeper soul for this brief lifetime and not our basic identity, then this radically changes our conception of who we are. The mystery of the psyche cannot be uncovered through outer means or through an introspection that fails to penetrate past the frontal self. Understanding of the self and psyche must come through a deepening inner vision of which only the spiritual traditions have been capable so far, an inner sight that extends all the way to our psychic center.

Toward an Integral View of the Self

Integral psychology sees the self as the centralizing function of the frontal consciousness. As the soul puts forth a body-heart-mind organism in each new human incarnation, it needs a way to organize the organism's experience into an integrated whole. There must be some central guidance process and command center, a way to integrate the body's perceptions and actions (the physical system), the heart's impulses and feelings (affective system), and the mind's thoughts and perceptions (cognitive system). All of these various data streams need to be synthesized into a coherent whole, otherwise we would never be able to get out of bed, let alone wash, get dressed, eat, work, interact, and function on many different levels throughout the day.

For the organism to survive and adapt it must centralize control, otherwise the body will pull in one direction, the heart in other directions, the mind in still others. The self acts both as a command center and as a guiding, orienting process, a center for coordination and synthesis of our internal needs and desires with our external perceptions and actions. The self coordinates the information flow from the three sheaths (*koshas*) of the body, heart, and mind. It not only processes information, it evaluates information and determines what action to take and so serves as the crucial executive function. The self is a developmental necessity, not just an accident or an illusion or the result of wounding. It centralizes consciousness on the surface.

Behind the self lies a deeper psychic center that gives the sense of identity or selfhood to the ego. The psychic center maintains contact with its surface instruments through the self. For the first stages of human evolution, this contact is minimal. The psychic center is young and less individualized, not strong or developed enough to exert significant control over the self and the frontal being. The self is almost completely run by its physical, emotional, and mental nature. As the psychic center develops further, however, it increases its influence and guides the self toward deeper values—truth, love, beauty, goodness, spirituality. However, this contact is on an inner plane and beyond the view of ordinary consciousness, hidden behind a veil, as Eastern psychology puts it.

The gradual growth of the psychic center and its purifying and refining effect upon the self proceeds without conscious awareness for a long period of time. As the refinement of the self proceeds, there is a greater inner and spiritual orientation, a magnetic attraction to the deeper sources of psychic life, as the inner dimensions of being start to open. The self becomes more translucent, more responsive to the promptings of the spiritual essence within. First the mind and the higher emotional parts turn toward a deeper life within and toward spirituality, but the frontal instruments are still accustomed to act on their own.

At some point the experience of the psychic center becomes conscious, and a new dimension of existence opens up. The psychic center is like a new organ of consciousness. It opens up a new dimension of awareness. At first this new perception is faint and unclear, though with time it gets stronger and more definite. At a later stage, the ego itself disappears, as the psychic center realizes its oneness with atman and comes forward to assume the executive functions of the instrumental being.[2]

Alain Grandcolas has researched the emergence of the psychic center or evolving soul in a number of individuals (Grandcolas, 2004.) There seem to be common elements in the experience of the psychic "bursting forth" from its egoic shell. These include the experience triggering "a sudden great joy without external cause," accompanied by "a strong feeling of love," and an awareness that "the individual harbours something immortal" within. Once the psychic "bursting forth" has occurred, it seems to remain a permanent part of consciousness in most individuals. Although Grandcolas discovered numerous individuals who have undergone the psychic "bursting forth," which may be likened to a hole being broken open in the shell of ego consciousness, he did not find anyone in his survey who experienced the full "coming to the front" of the psychic (which the Mother called a "reversal of consciousness"). The process of the soul coming to the front can be experienced as a gradual enlargement of the hole in the shell by which the psychic center's influence on the surface self becomes greater and greater. This enlargement of the hole indicates the process of psychic transformation (or psychicization).

At present, most human beings are identified with their frontal being. It is in this atmosphere that Western psychology has grown up—a nearly complete identification of the self with the instrumental nature. Though our identification with our frontal self and organism is almost total, most everyone has had some glimpses of the greater possibilities of our inner being. Freeing ourselves from this preoccupation with our frontal nature and finding our true identity are the key goals in integral psychology. It is not that our frontal self is not real, it is just superficial, the outermost covering of who we are.

Western psychology helps identify and engage with our self. It maps the self's powers and realms. It has captured the skeletal outlines of the self but not its flesh-and-blood or inner psychic essence. From the perspective of Western psychology, the self will always remain a mystery. As Kohut put it:

> The self . . . is . . . not knowable in its essence. . . . We can describe the various cohesive forms in which the self appears, can demonstrate the several constituents that make up the self . . . and explain their genesis and functions. We can do all that, but we will still not know the essence of the self as differentiated from its manifestations. (Kohut, 1977, pp. 310–312)

Kohut is correct, so far as he goes, but integral psychology goes farther. What animates the self, what gives it its distinctive individuality, is not simply the nuclear self (or Jung's "Self" or gestalt's "organism" or whatever we choose to call it). What is possible, even certain, at some point in our development is to directly experience the psychic center from which our self derives. This is our true individuality, our very soul and deepest self. Integral psychology provides a satisfying answer to the puzzle of selfhood, to what the inmost core of subjectivity is, the sense of being a being. Until we find and experience our psychic center, we will not know who we most truly are.

IMPLICATIONS OF THE PSYCHIC CENTER FOR PSYCHOLOGY

The deep psychic center is the evolutionary principle within us. Its upward evolutionary journey is reflected in the self it puts forth.

Growth and development are the essence of being human. The authentic self, in spite of its protective strategies and defensive impasses, is characterized by a relentless growth and expansion, a vital need to affirm itself, express itself, to expand beyond its limits.

Two lines of development are occurring: an outer line of the physical-emotional-mental self, which Western developmental psychology studies, and an inner line of psychic or soul development, to which Eastern traditions point. In studying the development of the frontal self, even this outer line of development cannot be fully understood without reference to the development of the psychic center and its progressive influence and refinement of the frontal being. As the psychic center develops in its unique way, it successively puts forth an expression of this uniqueness in each new incarnation. This becomes the essential nature (svabhava) from which the authentic self emerges. As the frontal ego progressively aligns with its deeper essential nature, this can become a path by which to realize its higher nature or psychic center and undergo a psychic, spiritual transformation. However, there are significant obstacles to this path of psychic realization.

Just as the light of the stars cannot be seen during the day because of the sun's overpowering light, so the inner light of our psychic center is initially difficult to see because of the brightness of our mind, emotions, and body. Until the glare of these frontal instruments is subdued, there is little chance of the psychic center's light getting through. The first task in all spiritual traditions is to dim the glare of the instrumental nature so the greater spiritual light can be seen. Integral psychology seeks not to extinguish these lights but to transform them so that first they will be responsive to the inner spiritual light and then themselves become instruments through which the soul's light may shine.

The movement toward the psychic center is open to all, natural, and in the course of evolution, inevitable. What is required is an aspiration and a sincerity of seeking, for it is through the heart's power that the inner being opens and the psychic light emerges. The mind alone, which is what we are most used to exercising, is helpless to affect this inner opening, although the mind's assent and will are necessary. We approach our psychic center most naturally through the heart, and it therefore becomes crucial to clear away the obstructions along the heart's path, which fall into two major categories:

- The fragmentation that results from the wounds, structural deficits, and defensive structures that make up so much of the unconscious. This universal psychological wounding is perhaps the single greatest obstacle that no spiritual tradition has yet been able to surmount on a large scale. A century of concerted effort by psychology has uncovered pieces of this puzzle that only now are we ready to synthesize into an integral whole. It needs to be considered first, because the difficulties it presents are so formidable that efforts to deal with the second category tend to be overpowered by it and easily degenerate into spiritual bypassing.
- The heaviness or obscurity of our consciousness that Eastern psychology and all spiritual practices work to purify. This will be taken up in ensuing chapters, along with how the two categories work together and can be clearly separated only on a conceptual level.

If psychology is to be a discipline that goes beyond the surface to include the full range of the psyche, then it must incorporate Eastern discoveries about human consciousness. Acknowledging that the deeper nature of psychic life is ultimately spiritual brings about a paradigm shift that fundamentally changes the field of psychology.

Chapter 3

The Core Wounding of Our Time

> . . . for that is the pressing need of the individual, to arrive at the highest
> truth of his own being, to set right its disorders, confusions, false identifica-
> tions, . . . to know and mount to its source.
> —Sri Aurobindo, *Synthesis of Yoga*

If our deepest identity is a joyous, loving, luminous center of peace, then why do we not experience this? Why in fact do we so often experience the very opposite?

Eastern psychology unambiguously declares that our deeper identity is veiled by the activity of the ego. This activity of the self kicks up so much dust that it clouds or obscures the inner light. Such obscurations as attachments and desires of all kinds pull us outward, and the ensuing fear, anger, stress, and emotional storms cover the deeper light and lull us to sleep. Until this activity is quieted and "purified," the light cannot get through, or at best it is glimpsed only in rare flashes.

Eastern traditions have considered impurity a single phenomenon, and spiritual practices are methods to quiet and purify the self. But spiritual practice works extremely slowly for most everyone. For a tiny few, spiritual practice succeeds magnificently, but religious traditions have been notably unsuccessful in bringing about a spiritual transformation in the world at large. The reasons for this become clear as we bring depth psychology to bear on this issue. An integral perspective reveals two different aspects to the self's "impurity":

53

1. Fragmentation or lack of integration of the self
2. Dense, heavy, "gross," or opaque consciousness

The problem with a purely spiritual approach to purification is that attempting to purify a fragmented self is a bit like trying to fill a sieve with water. A fragmented self works against itself, even in its spiritual practice. Spirituality works to refine the density or opacity of consciousness, but it is poorly equipped to deal with unconscious defenses and the self's fragmentation, for which it was never designed. Psychotherapy, on the other hand, was designed for and works to integrate the fragmented self, but it does not attempt to spiritualize or refine the consciousness, nor does it have the theoretical understanding by which to understand such an effort.[1]

The self, which centralizes consciousness and regulates affect, is also the result of innumerable wounds and unconscious defenses to cope with them. These wounds to the self are of paramount importance for inner development, because the fragmentation that results from this wounding makes any turning inward problematic. From infancy on, our senses pull us outward. We quickly become attached—to people, to emotional satisfactions, to mother's love and fear of disapproval, to physical pleasure such as nursing, eating, walking, moving, exploring. We soon develop a self that organizes our actions. As the self grows, desires and attachments multiply, drawing us out into the world. We come to identify with our surface body-heart-mind self and desires as we lose contact with our deeper nature.

We also are emotionally wounded in the process of development, and our attempts to cope with our wounding result in the growth of a dense underbrush of unconscious defenses against our emotional pain. The momentum of our turning away from our pain builds habitual attentional patterns over the years that eventuate in enduring psychological structures. Structures are psychological processes that abide, acting along repetitive grooves. When these neurological pathways are formed after much repetition, they become entrenched ways of coping that change only with concerted effort and under special circumstances of emotional arousal (such as depth therapy), otherwise they persist throughout one's lifetime. Getting through these unconscious defensive structures is something few people can do successfully through spiritual practice alone, except in sporadic flashes.

Our defenses work against inner deepening. The self has hidden from itself and becomes an unwitting victim of its own defensive maneuvers. Trapped in a web of its own making, it becomes hard to see more than a quarter inch below the surface, and the self has little chance of penetrating the still deeper veils that cover the psychic center. Whether a particular spiritual practice aims at opening the heart or greater mindfulness, the self is confined to a small circle, tethered to the unconscious defenses that prevent it from widening and deepening into the interior spaces of inner being.

So many obscurations are the result of fragmentation—incomplete gestalts, inhibitions, projections, fantasies and daydreams, self-manipulations, shoulds, shame, fear, guilt, obsessions—just what depth psychology studies in minute detail. What can we make of this tangle? How can it be straightened and clarified so that our deeper nature may shine through? It is here that Western psychology can be of great help.

Western psychology breaks new ground with its in-depth investigation into the nature of psychological wounding. Depth psychology has put psychological pain under the microscope, and over the past century a remarkably consistent picture has emerged of the self's development, its wounding, and the defensive strategies employed to cope with this pain.

The core wounding of our time is a rip in the very fabric of the self. This wounding tears apart the delicate formations of the self just as they are first forming, producing holes or gaps in the self's structure, blocking development in key areas, and disowning large portions of the self's experience that become unconscious and unavailable.[2] Dissociation from the body is the second major effect of wounding, and all of this is further exacerbated by trauma, which adds an additional push into dissociation, for dissociation is the defense of choice in trauma. Though clients who have been abused or traumatized often believe that trauma is the only problem, trauma is usually in addition to the pervasive structural wounds.

There are three major conceptual streams by which psychology understands this wounding and ensuing lack of integration, each of which contributes an important piece to the puzzle. They are the cognitive-behavioral schools, the psychoanalytic schools, and the humanistic-existential schools. While wounding is an extraordinarily complex phenomenon, the global outlines of wounding come into focus when informed by these three streams. Let us take each in turn.

The cognitive-behavioral schools of psychology have studied in great detail how our cognitions or thoughts have an important influence on how we feel. One aspect of fragmentation, with its concomitant depression, anxiety, and other painful feelings, is unrealistic, illogical thinking. Cognitive and behavioral therapists have discovered that bringing about better, more logical thinking can reduce such symptoms. For many people, this is sufficient. They are content to simply feel less pain and fewer symptoms and are not interested in inner deepening or a more complete working through. However, a change in thinking deals only with some of the most obvious surface manifestations of fragmentation, not the underlying causes. To understand the self's lack of integration it is necessary to consider how wounding is seen by the major streams of depth psychology—the psychoanalytic and the humanistic-existential.

STRUCTURAL-RELATIONAL DIMENSIONS OF CORE WOUNDING

Contemporary psychoanalysis views the self as emerging from early family relationships. Throughout life, the self is imbedded within a relational matrix that it needs for its ongoing nourishment and support. From the earliest moments of life to its end, the self requires a responsive environment of attuned people in order to thrive.

Different object relations schools and intersubjective and interpersonal schools are in wide agreement that a key aspect of psychological life is the self's ability to regulate its feelings and affects, with particular importance given to the needs to feel safe and free from anxiety. Classical self psychology (Kohut, 1971, 1977, 1984) adds three important lines of development: (1) an expansive sector of the self, out of which come our ambitions, (2) an idealizing aspect of the self that forms our ideals, and (3) an area of skills and talents by which our ambitions and ideals can be realized.

Kohut originally called the expansive pole the exhibitionistic-grandiose self, for this is how it presents itself in its earliest forms. Every child needs to feel wonderful and beloved—the fairest of them all—and looks to its parents as mirrors to confirm this greatness. If the main caretaker, usually the mother, is free enough of her own narcissistic concerns to look at the child with a gleam in her eye that says "You are an incredible child!," then this need can be met. Note that Kohut stresses that it is not the *words* of the mother that count here, it is the warmth in her eyes, her tone of voice, the *energy* with which she shows delight in her young child. Of course, even a theoretically perfect mother would be unable to provide this all of the time, but when occasional failures are not traumatic or overly intense, this "optimal frustration" allows the grandiosity to become modified, so that gradually the need to be the fairest of them all or perfect recedes, replaced by a solid feeling of self-worth. Internal structures of the self emerge during a slow developmental process that provides the person with healthy self-esteem and energizing ambition. This is the expansive dimension of the self.

A second need of the child is to feel that at least one parent, often the father, is calm, wise, strong, and powerful. Having contact with the idealized parent allows the child to partake of this calmness, strength, and power so that gradually these can be internalized as guiding ideals and self-soothing structures within the self. The prototype for an idealizing relationship is a parent picking up a crying child and soothing it, allowing the child to merge with the parent's calm and settling down. Again, over time, the child recognizes that its parents are not perfect and omnipotent, and if this perception is gradual and nontraumatic, then through internalization the person establishes the capacity to tolerate his or her own powerful feelings and impulses, to self-soothe, and to express or contain feelings as appropriate.

A third need of the self is to feel similar to other people, a person among other persons, an identification with someone with whom there is a likeness or similarity. This allows the child to feel part of the human community and to be encouraged in activities, paving the way for unfolding the innate skills and talents by which ambitions and ideals can be realized.

The development of the self and its potentials requires the world and human relationships to bring forth these capacities. Current trends in psychoanalysis emphasize the relational nature of the self and its need for nourishing relationships to sustain it throughout life. Contemporary self psychology emphasizes the functions that relationships play in facilitating a person to integrate affect, particularly those warded-off feelings and emotional experiences that are painful or fragmenting.

Ideally a child develops a cohesive self, in touch with ambitions, guiding ideals, and the skills and talents by which these ambitions and ideals can be realized, and the child is able to form relationships in which these aspects can be nurtured and brought forth. However, the world is far from this. Virtually everyone is born into a family in which there is deep wounding to the self. The average or normal self is not of one piece, cohesive and integrated. It is more like Swiss cheese, with numerous holes or deficits in the structure of the self. The result of countless "slings and arrows of outrageous fortune," the deficits in the self's structure are larger or smaller depending upon the type and timing of the injury, with developmentally earlier injuries having the greatest impact. Such a fragmentation-prone self can "fall apart" or fragment when slighted; this produces a disruption in the self's coherence, which we experience as lowered self-esteem, embarrassment, or humiliation.

The core wounding of our time results in a disruption of the coherence of the self, feelings of shame, and a sense of being intrinsically "bad," defective, or unlovable. Those affects and potentials most central to the self are the most vulnerable to wounding and shame. Unless they receive sustained, attuned, loving, and affirming nurturance (and every human being requires a good deal of this over long stretches of time), some degree of wounding is inevitable. According to affect theory and research (Nathanson, 1992; Tomkins, 1963), shame interrupts those affects that are most pleasurable and essential to the self, such as sexuality and the need for love, affirmation, and safety. Shame occurs when interest and excitement outstrip ability, which is why it can be experienced even in the first weeks of life, leading to a sense of a "defective self" (Nathanson, 1992.) It is a psychological version of "original sin."[3]

Shame is perhaps the most painful affect. Tomkins describes it like this:

> If distress is the affect of suffering, shame is the affect of indignity, of transgression and of alienation. Though terror speaks to life and death and distress makes of the world a vale of tears, yet shame strikes deepest into the heart of man. While terror and distress hurt, they are wounds inflicted from the outside which penetrate the smooth surface of the ego; but shame is felt as an inner torment, a sickness of the soul. It does not matter whether the humiliated one has been shamed by derisive laughter or whether he mocks himself. In either event he

feels himself naked, defeated, alienated, lacking in dignity and worth. (Tomkins, 1963, p. 118)

The greatest power of shame, however, comes later on as the self is developing amidst its interpersonal world. During the initial years in the development of the self, when the urgent needs for affirmation and love are intensely felt but empathically attuned, responses from the mother or caregiver are insufficient, shame is an inevitable outcome, leading to a sense of being "unloved and unlovable" (Wurmser, 1981).

This leads the self to fall from its developmental path and to adopt a false self that it hopes can be loved and affirmed. Shame precipitates our move into inauthenticity. By this move the child hopes to get back into the parents' good graces and to protect what cohesion is left. But by sacrificing our own authentic nature in the process, our self's defense against core wounding amounts to selling ourselves out, abandoning our true nature for a counterfeit image in order to maintain the lifeblood of ongoing parental approval. Shame causes us to separate from our original wholeness, to hide from ourselves (Broucek, 1991.) Shame highlights what we believe are failures, especially failures of the most vulnerable, central areas of the self. Our deepest sense of aliveness and excitement, the joy of being a being, and the most pleasurable dimensions of our self's experience are the most vulnerable to shame. As failures of emotional attunement are inevitable in the trial-and-error process of self-expression, shame becomes a universal component of the self's experience.

Shame is such an aversive feeling that we immediately avoid whatever feelings and parts of the self feel shameful. To keep shameful feelings at bay, anxiety and fear (which in affect theory are forms of the same affect) warn us when we are in danger of feeling ashamed. Freud's discovery of signal anxiety, which alerts the unconscious that unacceptable feelings are beginning to emerge, takes on new significance as the key to neurotic contraction and avoidance. Anxiety/fear and shame are the two primary affects that run the neurotic, defensive coping strategies used to shield us from our core wounding. However, these defensive coping strategies, in keeping so much of the authentic self cordoned off, fail to nourish and engage the full self. By reinforcing the inauthentic patterns designed to minimize anxiety and fear and shame, symptoms result, such as depression, stress, anxiety, addictions, intimacy and relationship problems, and so on. Generally only a concerted psychotherapeutic effort can overcome our tendency to stay away from shameful feelings to heal the wounding that shame covers.

Structural difficulties are reflected in problematic relationships. Without the wisdom and discernment of the authentic self, the wounded self recreates the dysfunctional relationship patterns of the original family. The imaginal capacities of the higher emotional get hijacked by the repressed, disavowed energies of the lower and central emotional and used for unconscious fantasy, profoundly influencing daily relationships. The use of the higher emotional's creativity to express the lower and central emotional forces—sexuality, power, aggression, self-esteem, and so on—results in a loss of the imaginal's role in receiving the inner being's higher inspirations. The creativity of our inner being is dimmed as creative capacity is channeled into the ego's ambitions, hopes, and fears.

The role of unconscious fantasy in organizing a person's life and relationships is a central discovery of psychoanalysis. Sometimes referred to as "organizing principles" (Stolorow, Brandchaft, & Atwood, 1987), our first family relationships lay down in the brain neural pathways that create prototypes for our relational world and are strengthened over time by repeated use. These emotional prototypes ("attractors") lead us to find potential lovers similar to the original attachment figures of mother and father. The unconscious pull of these attractors is unerring in locating conflicted, difficult relationships that are unfulfilling in old, familiar ways. Indeed, without a good deal of inner work, such relationships are about the only ones that are compelling and magnetic. In contrast, people who are truly loving and nourishing hardly even register on the radar. As a result, only a fraction of the intimacy and emotional nurturing that relationships can provide is ever developed, since so much of the self and its relational potential is "off-limits." Living in an interpersonal desert, it is just a short step to withdraw further from relationship and seek gratification in things, drugs, food, electronic entertainment, and compulsive activity.

Whereas in the West defects in the structure of the self are the result of isolation and lack of attuned contact, in the East the disturbances in the self's structure tend to be more related to impingements upon the self by family and society that do not allow the authentic self to emerge. This enmeshment and lack of clear boundaries submerge the authentic self and result in a false self that has a greater identification with the collective ego or group self of family and society. In the West the narcissistic wounding is the result of and results in isolation and estrangement from others; in the East the narcissistic wounding is the result of and results in enmeshment and failure to differentiate from others. While neither one is better or worse, the result is that both prevent the authentic self from emerging. A healthy, cohesive, and differentiated self can emerge and thrive in either cultural climate if family conditions are right. There is no "preferred" cultural condition for the self's development. Optimally, the diversity of cultures around the world would bring about different kinds of cohesive selves that result from widely varying self-other configurations.

In its wounded and defensively contracted state, the self looks very much like the fragmentation-prone self of contemporary psychoanalysis. Psychoanalytic theory beautifully depicts the self's struggle for cohesion amidst a malattuned family history and an interpersonally challenging present, but it has not recognized the embodied nature of the self and the larger organismic reality of the psyche. Psychoanalysis takes the culturally average dissociated state of an overly mentalized existence as normal rather than as a consequence of the self's wounding. As noted in earlier chapters, the early wounds bring not only repression and disavowal but dissociation from the body as well. The self leaves the body and retracts into the mind to cope with these early wounds, and the resulting fragmentation involves both a splintering of the self's structures *and* a separation of mind from body. It is here that the humanistic and existential approaches enlarge our view.

SOMATIC DIMENSIONS OF CORE WOUNDING

Wilhelm Reich was the first depth psychologist to chart the somatic roots of the self, and the myriad somatic therapies since then trace their lineage to his groundbreaking work. The rise of humanistic and existential schools of psychology derives from the powerful truth that we are a holistic body-heart-mind unity whose feeling life is embedded in the body. Further, our human organism is a source of innate intelligence. When the self aligns with its deeper organismic wisdom, we move naturally in the direction of actualizing our potentials and talents. Embodied life has profound depth and meaning when we open to the marvel of our organismic experiencing, in contrast to which the overly mentalized life of the average person seems relatively empty and shallow.

The humanistic and existential schools of depth psychology are in accord with psychoanalysis, that early experiences in the family are responsible for how the self develops, is wounded, and defends against those wounds, but they stress wounding's impact on our experience of the body. In an optimal family, the parents would empathically attend to the child's emotional hurts and provide support and soothing so that intense affects could be integrated. When this happens the child can assimilate and cope with even extremely painful and strong feelings and continue to sense these feelings as they stream throughout the body and come to their natural conclusion.

However, when the parents are not well attuned, as inevitably happens, the intensity of the feelings in the body causes the child to contract against this pain, to inhibit breathing in order to reduce the intensity, and to flee into the mind to escape such painful, overwhelming feelings. The child dissociates from uncontrollable bodily feelings into the mind, where there *is* more control. In so doing, the child maintains this contracted, retracted stance and braces against further injuries from this place of greater safety in the mind. Each new wounding further reinforces this stance, and soon it all becomes automatic, unconscious, and even seems natural, for it is a coping strategy that does work to reduce the strength of feelings.

However, as depth psychology has discovered, all defenses come at a price. And the price of leaving our body is vast and complex. The first consequence of dissociation comes as we contract our muscles against our pain. We squeeze ourselves, hold ourselves in, and tighten up against the distressing feelings in order to inhibit the flow of feeling within us. We literally get a grip on ourselves and then maintain that grip, even when we are safely out of danger and could relax. Contracting the muscles of the body, especially the deep muscles of the core, succeeds in deadening the intensity of feelings. However, when we relax this constriction, feelings begin to flow once again, usually starting with where they left off, and this is exactly what needs to be avoided. To ensure that these feelings are safely cordoned off, this bodily tension needs to be maintained. This eventuates in what Reich came to call the body armor, a system of chronically contracted muscles throughout the body that inhibits every facet of our feeling life and deadens bodily awareness.

The net result of this chronic inhibition is that we become rigid, uptight, and forever on guard against deep, intense feelings. Our feeling life is muted and suppressed as we work to reduce our own aliveness. We become neurotically deliberate and lose the spontaneity of living. This also amounts to a terrible waste of energy as we work against ourselves, protect ourselves from our own feelings and impulses by pushing down the very life energy that enlivens us.

Concurrent with contracting against our feelings comes holding our breath. Excitement and strong feelings require metabolic support to uphold them. Just as fire needs oxygen to burn brightly, so the body's energetic aliveness depends upon oxygen to maintain it. Breathing freely occurs naturally in infants as the breath changes constantly in response to the baby's interests and excitement. Contracting our muscles and inhibiting our breathing are the two main ways that feelings are suppressed and eventually repressed. Holding our breath reduces the intensity of feelings, and over time this strategy also becomes chronic and habitual. With it also comes a reduction of our entire feeling capacity, for it is a truism that "You can't go higher than you can go low." Restricting the intensity of painful affects has the unwanted side effect of restricting the intensity of pleasurable feelings as well.

REPRESSION, DISAVOWAL, DISSOCIATION

While primitive defenses such as denial, splitting, and projection are favored in severe psychological disorders, in the normal neurosis of our time the major defenses that an injured self utilizes are repression, disavowal, and dissociation. Repression keeps the early, frustrated needs down and away from consciousness. Disavowal keeps the self from acknowledging the importance of important relationships. Dissociation removes the self from the intensity of bodily reality as it retreats into the mind. Begun and reinforced in the family of origin, there is great pressure to protect both the parents and the child by minimizing the impact of painful and conflictual interactions. The family engages in a conspiracy of silence not to speak about the feelings with which the parents have difficulty or by which they are embarrassed. Children need a supportive relationship that will help them identify, tolerate, express, and integrate their feelings; without this, children quickly learn to pretend that certain interactions do not have an emotional impact or to hide this impact from others and from themselves.

Growing up in such an environment teaches the child to disavow feelings and the impact of other people in all settings. As the child ventures out into the world, it appears as if the whole of society is engaged in a vast conspiracy of silence, for there are very few places where it is safe to acknowledge deep feelings or express them freely. As psychology's influence permeates the larger society, this is slowly changing, but the shame over feelings still takes a heavy toll on every individual.[4]

One consequence of disavowal as an ongoing defense is not recognizing the immense importance of our relationships for psychological health. People grow up not knowing their interpersonal needs, hardly realizing that they have these needs. Psychology has contributed to this by its insistence, during its first 75 years on independence and autonomy, on a belief that being dependent on others was bad or indicated psychopathology. This is still a popular view of healthy independence held by many people. However, contemporary depth psychology has radically altered its first views of independence and now sees clearly just how deeply dependent or interdependent everyone is. Life is a team sport. The self exists in a relational matrix of important relationships. When too isolated or estranged from this relational matrix, the self fragments or "falls apart."

We live in a time where most people experience only a small fraction of the power and beauty of intimacy. The richness of emotional connection, the deeply meaningful union with others, the depths of love and the emotional seas it is sometimes necessary to cross to come upon these depths, and the infinite variety of relationships and the new parts of ourselves evoked in them reveal dimensions of relationships that wounding and its defenses make off-limits.

In the West this produces a fragmentation-prone self that is beset with shame, anxiety, depression, and stress, preoccupied with its own competence, fearful in relationships, and rarely capable of true intimacy, alienated from its own deeper self, committed to an inauthentic life of distraction and entertainment, addictions, and pseudo-intimacy, with at best sporadic periods of feeling emotionally nourished by relationships or work. In the East disavowal results in a fusion of self and culture. Fear of alienating family, friends, or coworkers causes the self to be submerged by the needs of the group. This eventuates in a failure to differentiate and realize the fullness of individuation that is possible. In the West the failure of individuation produces a pseudo-independent, fragmented self divorced from its authentic depths. In the East the failure of individuation produces an enmeshed self that also is divorced from its authentic depths.

In dissociating from the body, we lose touch with our natural functions: breathing, speaking, sexuality, eating, moving, sensing. We squeeze our voice so that it becomes constricted, shrill, higher, and more forced than when we are relaxed and more deeply centered. Since breathing is restrained, our capacity for sexual excitement also is reduced. The intensity of pleasure that we can tolerate, the power of breathing to support sexual arousal, the freedom of the body to move and the pelvis to swing freely in supporting and building sexual feelings, the ability to vocalize freely, the strength of orgasm, and even the degree of relaxation afterward are affected by this overarching inhibition.

In moving from the body to the mind, we also leave behind the immense richness of the sensory world. Part of the wonder of childhood is the intensity and awe of drinking in the world through our eyes, ears, and body. Our sensory awareness is our most fundamental reality. Taking in the beauty of nature's sights and sounds, feeling the joy of our body moving in space in even simple activities such as walking or reaching up in the cupboard for a glass, really seeing the people we talk to, feeling the softness of the skin in our hand as we walk a child across the street—our life is a sensory feast. But in becoming addicted to the mind, thinking and fantasy replace sensing. "Lose your mind and come to your senses," Fritz Perls counseled. The average person today is lost in a fantasy world of thinking, planning, rehearsing, chewing over unfinished situations from the past, and imagining future triumphs, immersed in the past and future but lost to the present moment. In losing the present moment, we lose presence; we are only "half there," no longer fully engaged in our actual, living experience.

Another facet of overly mentalized living is losing awareness of how our feelings live in the body, how they stream through us in a physical way. Feelings cannot be reduced to body sensations, for even athletes and those who are physically active are generally typically unconscious of feelings. But the capacity to sense our feelings is part of our embodied existence. Through dissociation we lose touch with our felt sense and the ever-moving stream of our physical-emotional experiencing. On a more subtle level, we also lose touch with our life energy and the subtle physical underpinnings of the body. The process of tightening up and holding ourselves down has the effect of shutting off more subtle levels of perception. This coarsening of perception blunts our sensitivity and keeps us from sensing more refined energies in our body and environment.

Emotional-physical suppression affects the subtle body and energy field, which then has a direct effect on physical health as well. Chronic inhibition and emotional repression result in immune suppression, as the new mind-body field demonstrates (see, e.g., Pert, 1997, 1998; Goleman & Gurin, 1993). The fact that greater disease susceptibility is linked to the unconscious, defensive processing of emotions has immense implications for health, which is only now being explored.

Eating is another casualty of leaving the body. In abandoning the body, in place of body awareness we have a hole, an inner emptiness, and food is one way of filling it. Yet this divorce from the body makes it hard to even sense when we are full, so the body's own self-regulating system is thrown out of kilter. Eating itself becomes something else to control, and in trying to control eating, the self ends up *being controlled* by emotional pressures. Food becomes used for emotional regulation, a way to calm down, numb out, and deaden the constant uptightness created by chronic contraction, which then requires stimulants to offset it. Living in the mind, we hardly even taste or smell our food. We become alienated from chewing, a basic avenue by which we take in nourishment. Instead, we seek foods that are easy to swallow. The rise of fast food in the culture points to how deeply alienated so many are from the function of eating. Attempts to control eating alternate with out-of-control binges that are hard for the person to understand when attempts to dominate the body backfire and the body revolts.

The net effect of dissociation is a self and culture that are disconnected from the natural world, life out of balance. While it is important to realize that we are more than our body, defensive dissociation is neither integration nor spiritual detachment; it is alienation. In losing touch with our functions of breathing, eating, sexuality, speaking, and moving, these become fragments of our total self. Cut out of the context of relatedness, they become isolated, compartmentalized, and objectified. Our body becomes a thing to be dominated, like everything physical—animals, the planet, women, native peoples—another indication of estrangement from our full being. When we no longer feel the depths of our bodily reality, we are uprooted from our ground. This dissociation is essential to heal for an integral living.

The spiritual consequences of wounding are far-reaching. More than anything else, the defenses against our wounding close our heart. Through repression, disavowal, dissociation, and other defenses we lose our inborn openness and vulnerability. We abandon our heart and flee into a fantasy world of mental images. We harden our hearts to stop feeling our own pain and to protect ourselves from being wounded again. A closed heart diminishes love, compassion, and mindfulness.

A major dimension of spiritual purity is consciousness of our own narcissism. When narcissistic wounding is unconscious, the pain of this trauma, the archaic, unmodified grandiosity that has been disavowed, and the consequent defects in the self's structure seriously retard spiritual development. When spiritual experience does break through, it tends to be captured by the unconscious narcissistic demands and used for ego inflation and self-aggrandizement. Primitive grandiosity is, in one sense, impurity itself, for it feeds egoism and claims for the ego what is the Divine's. So much of the spiritual marketplace today is a result of this—teachers who have had passing experiences or minor realizations that are then taken over by archaic grandiosity and narcissistic demands. Without a good deal of psychotherapeutic work to heal the narcissistic wounding so that a more mature, modulated, healthy sense of self-esteem can develop, unmodified grandiosity remains unconscious and blocks further spiritual development.

Wounding and its attending defenses limit mindfulness by keeping so much of the self's experience off-limits and unconscious. Mindfulness works well to bring awareness to the physical body and breath, but it has a very limited effect on bringing out the emotional dimension and undoing defenses such as repression, disavowal, and dissociation. For this reason Buddhist practice aims at first opening the heart through devotional (*metta*) practices, but here again such practices have little effect on the defensive structure. It is the same problem theistic traditions face with devotional or bhakti practices. They tend to be limited to the higher emotional realm and hardly touch the central emotional or lower instinctual emotional levels of everyday life. The self, with its unconscious needs, grabs the heart's aspiration and twists it to its own narcissistic ends.

A fragmentation-prone self is preoccupied by its self-image and with how others see it, so there is a continual pull outward into interpersonal anxiety and stress that prevents the calm and peace so necessary for spiritual deepening. This is why so many spiritual practices leave relationships and the world behind, so that they will not distract the seeker from the central spiritual aim. However, on a path of integral transformation, such a strategy only avoids the problem rather than solves it.

Spiritual bypassing, which is the use of spiritual ideas and images to bolster psychological defenses, is unavoidable for most without a good deal of psychological awareness. The neurotic separation of the mind from the body and feelings is bolstered by world-shunning philosophies that counsel a spiritual retreat from the world to a heaven or nirvana. Spiritual bypassing makes virtues of defensive detachment and dissociation. In an integral approach, this dissociation needs to be healed, and the body and feelings need to be owned. True detachment follows from owning, but it is unhealthy when it bypasses it.

It is not possible to enumerate all of the spiritual obstacles created by the narcissistic and somatic dimensions of wounding, just as all of the psychological sequelae are too numerous to detail, but so many have their sources in this area. Even those obstacles that are more a function of the density or murkiness of consciousness are further obscured by unconscious defenses. All forms of unconsciousness have darkening and lowering effects on consciousness. Anything of an inner nature—higher or deeper—passes through the self to reach the ordinary surface consciousness. The self seizes on and funnels all experience through its distorting, defensive processes. Until integration and coherence are brought to the self, this fragmentary action will disperse the inner light in a thousand directions.

In summary, core wounding affects every level of the self:

- Inner conflict as the self does battle with itself, dividing itself into conscious and unconscious sectors
- Mind—distorted, illogical thinking as mental clarity is sacrificed to defensive cognitions
- Higher emotional—loss of imaginal capacity, constriction of imagination and fantasy life as it gets channeled into daydreaming, erosion of ideals, less openness to inner planes
- Central emotional—disavowal, fragile or low self-esteem, difficulty finding nourishing relationships, anxiety, depression,

alienation, crippled capacity for intimacy, failure to find true, creative work
- Lower emotional—repression, inhibition of sexual and aggressive feelings, low vitality
- Body—dissociation and retreat to an etheric, disembodied mind state, loss of realness and sensory vividness, impaired immunity and health, reduced physical energy
- Reduced coherence of the self's integrity and coherence, loss of authentic self and relationships, development of a false self that covers up or compensates for wounds and deficiencies
- Spirit—fragmentation that makes inner deepening extremely difficult

Therapists of different orientations stress parts of this wounding proper to their own school, for example, a classical Freudian will emphasize the loss of instinctual energies, a Jungian will emphasize the loss of imaginal capacities, a relational therapist will focus on structural deficits and relational impairments, a somatic therapist will focus on dissociation from the body, and so on. But in all of this the path of healing leads through these two stages—the structural/relational and the somatic—before the psychological transformation culminates in the emergence of the authentic self.

This is a good beginning and is entirely sufficient for many people, but it leaves out our higher possibilities. It leaves the authentic self in the dark, guided only by its own reflected light. The authentic self only approximates wholeness; it comes close to it but cannot fully embody it, for true wholeness means an opening to our psychic center and spiritual ground. The psychic center is wholeness unalloyed. Psychological work leads up to psychic awakening, but stops short of it. The psychic opening is needed to complete and fulfill it, which takes us into areas of growth and transformation that are little known.

Chapter 4

An Evolutionary Vision of Health

> The coming of a spiritual age must be preceded by the appearance of an
> increasing number of individuals who are no longer satisfied with the
> normal intellectual, vital and physical existence of man but perceive that a
> greater evolution is the real goal of humanity.
> —Sri Aurobindo, *The Human Cycle*

The healing of the many levels of our early wounding, accompanied by
an increasingly authentic life, brings us to the highest potentials envisioned by Western psychology. Yet to stop here is to stop far short of
our human possibilities. From an integral perspective, the evolution of
consciousness entails two lines of development—an outer, surface line,
where a new body-heart-mind develops each new lifetime, and an
inner, soul line, where the psychic center develops over many lifetimes.

The evolution of consciousness is the central feature of psychological life.
All of psychology must be seen against this backdrop of evolving consciousness.[1] Out of all our difficulties and trials, frustrations and
achievements, confusions and bafflement, even through apparent failures and disappointments, we are developing a greater, deeper, higher
self. Hidden at first but then progressively sensed and felt, this deeper,
truer center unfolds ever-greater powers and abilities, extending and
deepening our capacities for feeling, thinking, willing, acting, and creating. It is the goal of integral psychology to align with the cosmic
evolutionary impulse as fully as we can to unfold our potentials.

This perspective has two implications:

1. *Developing our instruments is the goal of embodiment.* The growth of our body, heart, and mind is necessary for the fullness of living (a focus of Western psychology).

2. *Finding our evolutionary center is key.* Discovering the evolutionary element within us brings forth life's evolutionary guidance, a light that illumines our way amidst the darkness of the world (a focus of Eastern psychology).

Integral psychology seeks to do both: to develop our physical-emotional-mental self so it is a coherent, integrated expression of our authentic being (psychological transformation) and to find our psychic center so it becomes a guiding influence in our life (psychic transformation).

Integral psychology sees an inseparable interplay between these two dimensions. The psychic center is less developed in the initial stages of human evolution, where the emphasis is on developing the outer instruments, but as evolution proceeds, the deeper psychic center becomes stronger and more insistent, and it draws our attention inward. In moving consciousness beyond the superficial life on the surface, the depth dimension of the psyche opens to an inexhaustible richness and beauty. Psychology has not known how to go deeper than the self, and spiritual practice has not known how to work through the unconscious defenses and blocks that result from emotional wounding. An integral working includes both in our next evolutionary steps.

One of the great paradoxes, and one of the hardest for the human mind to accept, is the growth of consciousness through the opposites: from initial unconsciousness we find greater consciousness; through loneliness we realize the importance of others; out of brokenness and fragmentation we come upon wholeness; in pain and suffering the hard walls of the heart melt, and we open to love and joy; in the depths of shame can be found self-acceptance; in the darkness of hitting bottom we discover a redeeming light that raises us; in working through and deconstructing the false self we create an authentic life. As hard to bear as our wounding is, within it lie the seeds of our fulfillment.

THE SACRED WOUND

We are so used to thinking of our hurts and wounds only as a source of pain and trouble, yet gems of incalculable value are found in the heart of our darkness and pain. Our wounding, if we have eyes to see it, is a gift, wrapped in the dark camouflage of tears and suffering but containing the precious jewels of our salvation.

The world wounds everyone born into it. No one escapes life's blows. These blows hammer the ego's primal narcissism and grandiosity that claim for itself what belongs to the Divine. To defend against these blows the self defensively contracts and hardens. It develops only partially behind the shielding it erects to protect from future blows. The self, contracted and stunted, develops a false self as a coping strategy but becomes estranged from its authentic source.[2] However, this self is not entirely false. It is an amalgam of primary, authentic structure and defensive, false structure. This mixture of real and false composes the normal self. Psychological symptoms and suffering are signals that the self has been thrown off course.

Our symptoms and pain, much as we are ashamed of them and want them to go away, are stepping-stones to finding ourselves and unfolding our potentials. Symptoms result from the self disowning its own experience. The self wages a battle against itself, trying to cut itself off from itself. But disowned portions of the self do not just go away. They remain in the unconscious, continually seeking expression, which in turn demands continual, ongoing defense against them. This defensive process is never completely successful, and these disowned feelings leak out, pushing and pulling us toward people and activities that then create symptoms.

As noted earlier, wounding affects all levels of the self—somatic, lower, central, and higher emotional, mental. What depth therapy has discovered is that our pain is not something meaningless or useless to feel. Rather, when we fully embrace our suffering and reexperience the early feelings that our symptoms activate, our healing becomes a path for bringing forth buried parts of the self, allowing us to feel real once again, this time no longer as a mostly unconscious child but now as a more fully self-conscious adult.

HEALING, GROWTH, AND TRANSFORMATION

As used in this book, *healing* is a reparative process of working through old wounds and emotional hurts and trauma. *Growth* is the emergence of something new, new potentials unfolding, new feelings, new experiences, new parts of the self coming forth toward actualization. *Transformation* occurs when there is enough healing and growth to bring about the emergence of a new organizing principle that alters our entire being.

Beneath most old wounds lie new aspects of the unrealized self, dormant potentials that await healing and integration. Psychotherapy brings this buried self back on-line so its energies may enliven and enhance our life. However, this new growth does not emerge fully developed. It undergoes a process of maturation and development in which the new self's structure is built little by little, as small increments of growth consolidate over time. The new self's structure, like all new growth, is generally vulnerable and fragile, like new sprouts that tenderly reach up toward the light. Just as a greenhouse supports plants at first, so a safe, emotionally nourishing atmosphere (such as a therapeutic relationship) helps ensure that the self's new structures and growth are not uprooted and blown away by the world's jarring energies. After a period of development, these parts of the self become stronger and better able to withstand the world's forces. Our psychological wounds are the greatest impediment to our growth. Healing our wounds sets the stage for new growth, but growth must reach a critical mass before it becomes transformation.

Although most people want immediate transformation, there are no such sudden miracles. Transformation takes time. For example, the psychological transformation from normal neurosis to having the real, authentic self as the foundation of the psyche involves years of healing and growth to work through the false self formed in the person's family of origin.

In the spiritual realm, Sri Aurobindo was the first to point out the differences between *experience, realization,* and *transformation,* which are often confused with each other. Experiences come and go. Spiritual *experience* is a temporary entry into a spiritual state. It prepares the consciousness for a new level of realization, but it is not itself that new level. *Realization* is a permanent shift into a new realm of being, however, it leaves the outer nature relatively untouched. Much religious teaching is aimed at realization, an inner freedom but with the outer nature (*prakriti*) left to the momentum of its past karma. Many religious traditions maintain that transformation of this earthly nature is impossible, so that only when the body drops at death can there be total freedom. However, integral yoga holds that realization can extend to an entire transmutation of our outer nature, including the very cells of our body. When the power of the inner realization infuses and transmutes the outer nature, this is *transformation*. Realization is an inner attainment, but transformation changes our entire being, both inner and outer.

In the traditional path of realization there is no need to expand the self's capacities, because the self itself is seen as an impediment to be transcended rather than as an instrument to be developed. But in the integral path of transformation, our instrumental nature of body, heart, and mind is important—every level of our being that we are developing in this lifetime. In following the path of transformation, our ordinary life becomes the field for our development. Our relationships, our work, our play, our mating, fighting, fearing, and loving become the basis for our deeper unfolding. Rather than life leading away from the path, life becomes the path.

TWO TRANSFORMATIONS

An evolutionary vision of health starts with the unifying principle of *svabhava*. Health emerges from our authentic nature.[3] Pathology, disease, and disorder are expressions of fragmentation and inauthentic being. Health, healing, whole, holistic, holy—it is no accident that all of these words come from the same root. Health is an expression of wholeness, at whatever level of our being—physical health, emotional health, and mental health. As every person born becomes wounded, fragmented, and inauthentic to some degree, there is some amount of imbalance and pathology that comes with each incarnation. Similarly, the urge for healing and wholeness is an evolutionary urge felt by all, for it is inherent in the very nature of embodiment. Integral psychology sees two dimensions of this movement toward wholeness: a psychological transformation and a psychic transformation.

The Psychological Transformation

Western psychology charts the possibilities for psychological health at each level of the self. These health values reflect the highest possibilities envisioned by the different schools of psychology. Generally they are presented in isolation, each school declaring its own, level-specific view of psychological health. An integral view unites these disparate potentials into a unified whole.

Mind: At the level of mind, health consists in the capacity to think clearly, logically, and critically, without cognitive distortions, illogical reasoning, or irrational beliefs.

Higher emotional: Health at this level involves creativity, a rich fantasy life, intuition, and an openness to the imaginal realm and spiritual impulses. Creativity is not confined to painting a picture or producing a work of art but is an outflow from the depths of inner being. It can infuse everyday life and relationships as well as work and activities.

Central emotional: Health at this level involves a cohesive self inwardly and nourishing, loving relationships outwardly. Inner cohesion is expressed by a glow of healthy self-esteem and wholeness. Creative work where the person's true abilities, passion, and purpose converge is another hallmark of authentic selfhood. Genuine relationships of all kinds round out the central emotional. Some key forms authenticity takes are relationship with a lover; with family, close friends, and trusted colleagues with whom we can relax and be ourselves as well as with whom we can be vulnerable and intimate; and with mentors, guides, and teachers we respect and look up to.

Lower emotional: Here health takes the form of healthy sexuality, healthy aggression and self-assertiveness, and the enjoyment of the instinctive side of our nature.

Physical: Health at this level means a vivid sense of embodiment, not dissociated or disconnected from our physical being but alive to the sensory world and the beauty of nature; a body that is healthy, vital, and relaxed rather than contracted and uptight; a sense of rootedness in physical being with breathing freely supporting the energetic excitement of our feeling life coursing through our body.

When these health potentials become actualized, a state of integration results, or to use the vocabulary of neuroscience, *coherence.* Coherence means to hold together, to hang together, or cohere together. Just as a laser beam consists of coherent light waves that move together over great distances versus a beam of conventional light that disperses quickly, so psychological coherence produces a shimmering vibration of energy that is harmonious and concordant. What unifies the different parts of our being is our authentic nature (our *svabhava*), so our body, heart, and mind vibrate to a similar wavelength and create a harmonious self-expression that is consonant with our essential nature, rather than the jagged, dissonant, jarring, incoherent vibration of fragmentation.

Western psychology has produced a very precise map of our physical-emotional-mental self, and each school of psychology contributes to the healing, growth, and transformational possibilities of each level. Integral psychology synthesizes these insights into a larger whole that embraces each part of our being and raises them up to their highest potentials. However, as we progressively recognize, even the most fully developed, coherent self, no matter how actualized and fulfilled it may be, is still lost in the darkness of surface, fragmentary living. Full, integral living requires plunging still more deeply inside to find our psychic center. Even at its best, psychological wholeness is only a partial and diminished figure of wholeness. But spirit is wholeness itself. Spirit is the very principle of wholeness that puts forth this outer body-heart-mind. Psychological wholeness derives from this underlying spiritual wholeness. The psychological experience of selfhood is the experience of a fragment seeking wholeness.

The psychological transformation is a first approach to wholeness. We get glimpses of it in psychological states of coherence—states of flow and full engagement, states of authenticity and integration, states of deep intimacy and resonance with others, or communion with nature. Such states provide previews into the greater possibilities of wholeness that evolution is moving us toward. But such previews become a permanent reality only as we awaken to our psychic center and it comes forward.

The Psychic Transformation

Here we come upon new, evolutionary, emergent territory that is just beginning to be manifested. Putting health values in an evolutionary context reveals that psychological health changes as the outer, psychological nature spiritualizes. As the psychic flame in the heart burns brighter, the outer self refines and transforms. An inner consciousness opens, lighting up our outer nature. When the psychic center progressively exerts its influence, the course of our life changes, bringing us into contact with what we need for our growth—teachers, books, relationships, work, experiences. Challenges and adversity continue to be there, for difficulties come to all. But the ups and downs yield in the end to a dawning of the psychic light.

First comes the *awakening* of the psychic center, its realization as a frequent or constant part of our inner consciousness. The second step is the *coming forward* of our psychic center. As the soul comes to the front, the psychic consciousness begins to infiltrate our normal consciousness, permeating it with its light, joy, peace, discernment, love for all creation, gratitude, devotion, and aspiration. This psychic transformation brings forth the inner soul qualities into our surface being. Psychicization transmutes every level of the self. It is an infusion of soul force and soul consciousness that uplifts our outer nature and makes it a fitting instrument of Spirit. What does the psychic transformation look like?

Mind: The psychic transformation of mind brings a deep, vast peace and quietude to mind's incessant noise. Thought is not just more logical but becomes more intuitive, more luminous, more God centered and God focused. Greater mindfulness comes as we wake up to the present moment.

Higher emotional: Transforming this level means opening ever more to the spiritual, inner realms. Creativity becomes more linked to revealing visionary experience and appreciation of the all-beautiful Spirit in all of its manifestations. A growing need in our depths for beauty in our lives, a growing awe of the immense beauty of nature, and aesthetic experiences of beauty and delight permeate our daily experience.

Central emotional: As the psychic center's joy, love, and self-existent bliss are increasingly felt within, our relationships with others transform. As we appreciate just how relational we are, we find greater joy and fulfillment in relationships, together with greater recoil from those who are harsh and insensitive. In opening to an inner source of joy and an inner relationship with the Divine, our reliance on others diminishes (but does not end—trying to do so results in one kind of spiritual bypassing). Relationships that do not have a spiritual or psychic basis, those with only a mental, vital, or physical tie, are less energized and tend to lessen, whereas relationships with fellow seekers or spiritual community—*sangha*—become more important. Authenticity in relationships becomes even more valued, and when instilled with a psychic touch such relationships become priceless soul-to-soul connections. There is more love, more light, and more joy inwardly brought into relationships. The psychic consciousness brings greater sensitivity, empathy, sweetness, and tenderness into all contacts. A loving connection to all people and nature exists on an inner level, even though on an outer level there may be conflict and discord.

The psychic change brings about a shift in the self's equilibrium. The psychic center's inherent wholeness, joy, and fullness of being begin to permeate the self. Questions of self-esteem, whether high or low, arise less and less and then hardly at all, for this is a state complete in itself. This does not substitute for the healing and growth of the self but fulfills it and brings it to its acme.

Lower emotional: Here anger and aggression refine to become Force, an Energy or a Power to be used when needed. It is a power of assertion that becomes freer from hostility. Here the teachings of the *Gita* become more understandable, where Krishna tells Arjuna to fight powerfully but with a mind filled with peace and love.

The energies of sexuality may develop in several directions. One is the traditional way of sublimation, where sexuality is channeled into spiritual practice, used to elevate the consciousness rather than being thrown outward. A second direction lies along the path of Tantra, where sexuality becomes a form of worship and devotion. India's discovery of Tantra is unique in the world's spiritual traditions, for it provides a positive model of sacred sexuality along with information on how to use the energies of sexuality in the service of spiritual development. Here lovemaking becomes an electric meeting of souls, a devotional yoga involving body, heart, mind, and spirit. Rather than drawing away from sexual passion, these energies are harnessed and used for consciousness development. It may be that for most people, both of these directions will be used, both conserving energy and, when expressed, channeling it toward devotion, worship, and opening the heart.

Physical: The body senses changes in two directions. There is an increasing sense of the body being just a fringe on the surface, a superficial part of us. At the same time, there is an expansion of the body feeling into an immense depth, as we open up to its foundation in the subtle body. We come to experience the body as energy, and there is often a movement from purely physical exercise to forms of subtle physical exercise, such as yoga, aikido, tai chi, or qi gong. The bliss of the energy body comes with a sense of lightness and vitality, and the mystery of embodiment opens up new depths of profundity.

Spiritual: Unveiling the soul within reveals a fount of light, bliss, love, and peace that does not depend on any outer circumstances. The psychic center progressively infuses the outer self, refining its density and heaviness, so the outer being becomes responsive to the inner soul. The opening or awakening of the psychic center generally takes many years to come forward, as its transforming light slowly raises the outer being to a higher level.

The psychic transformation takes up each strand of our being— body, heart, and mind—and refines their energies, infusing each part with the psychic vibration and consciousness. The dross and impurities are slowly burned away. The grossness and heaviness of the body consciousness are refined so that its dense, apparent unconsciousness awakens and becomes lighter, subtler, raised to a finer vibration, sensitive to the subtle physical energies of the energy body. The energies of the emotional—lower, central, higher—are uplifted and infused with the love, joy, and peace of the psychic center. The *rajasic* vehemence of the emotional, its brash impulsivity and insistent, demanding sense of entitlement, is calmed, softened, and ennobled by the psychic's energies, purified so that the sensitivity of the emotional consciousness can be receptive to the inner promptings. The mind's self-assurance and arrogance are clarified and elevated, quieted so that in peace and silence the mind may receive true inner guidance.

The refinement of the psychic transformation changes each part of us, slowly or quickly as our nature demands and as the opening proceeds. The less integration of the self, the more it is divided into conflicting sectors, the more difficult it is to awaken the psychic and for the psychic influence to refine the self. Upsurges of vital desire and emotional storms of all kinds seize the self, throwing it into outwardness and deflecting it from its focus on awakening the true soul and psychic center. On the other hand, the greater the integration and coherence of the frontal self, the more readily the psychic influence and transformation can proceed.

COHERENCE, REFINEMENT, RESONANCE

Coherence is the result of the psychological transformation, a growing state in which increasing integration of the self's levels vibrate together, in harmony with the authentic nature native to the person. This greater coherence also brings about greater physical health and immune capacity, as recent medical advances document. Coherence is built upon authenticity, which extends into our relational world. It is a positive spiral of greater health, good feeling, and richness and fulfillment in work and relationships.

Refinement is the result of the psychic transformation, an evolving purification of the outer nature and self, bringing forth the inner qualities of the psychic center—peace, light, bliss and utter contentment, discrimination, gratitude, truthfulness, purified devotion and surrender, and openness to spirit. The surface instruments become more receptive to the inner source of consciousness, more loving, and more in touch with the inherent delight of being.

Coherence and refinement bring with them a third treasure—an increased capacity for resonance. The more coherent the self, the greater its capacity for resonance with others (Siegal, 1999). Resonance is pulsation at the same level, a sympathetic vibration in which we respond from similar parts of our being. In resonance we enter into an empathic immersion and depth of relatedness with another; together we participate in being. Resonance is a form of communication between two people, a form of sharing. Sometimes this is limited to the verbal level, but at its highest, we are able to resonate emotionally, mentally, and somatically, communing with one another at every level. It is true meeting and touching. A person's capacity for resonance with others is limited by the degree of coherence the self has achieved. A relatively less coherent self has significant limitations around intimacy and the capacity for resonance with others. Greater coherence brings with it the delight and fulfillment of deep capacity for resonance with others.

This capacity for resonance with others is not restricted to people—the other can be nature, animals, flowers, the natural world, music, or art. Resonance is the ability to be touched deeply, to be open and vulnerable and responsive to the reverberations of the world around us. The more fully we can be touched, the greater our fulfillment in life and relationships.

As the psychic transformation proceeds, it becomes clear that our capacity for resonance and deep intimacy with others is limited only by our connection to ourselves. We can only go as deeply with another as we can go into ourselves. Greater coherence on the personality level opens up immensely the potential for intimacy with others. However, even here it is still limited by the degree of sympathetic vibration that two distinct personalities can achieve. When we awaken our psychic center, the possibilities for deep intimacy expand infinitely, for we feel a oneness with all at the level of Being. Thus we get the example of great souls with an awakened psychic center, such as Jesus Christ, who related to all people, including the outcasts and the dark side of humanity—lepers, prostitutes, the insane—at the level of spirit or Being.

We sense an inner resonance and loving vibration—even if, at the level of personality, there is dissonance, discord, or even conflict. So while Krishna enjoins Arjuna to fight and destroy the enemy with a mind at peace and a heart full of love, on the inner plane there is peace, love, and light, even in the midst of war and destruction outwardly. Such a poise of consciousness creates the best chance for harmony and peace, but even if conflict or war is unavoidable, it can be carried out skillfully and mindfully. And when, instead of war, loving and intimacy are the goal, then how much more can be realized with the psychic center as the basis?

One of the great insights into the nature of reality that comes out of the schools of India Tantra is that all existence is vibration (*spanda*). Each particle, rock, blade of grass, planet, and star is a form of vibration. Embodiment in this manifest world is a vibratory adventure. From an integral perspective, evolution is a movement from a simple to a progressively more complex vibrational state. Greater complexity has the potential both for greater and more varied forms of dissonance (discord and unhappiness) as well as for greater and more varied forms of coherence (harmony and joy). Health is a coherent vibrational state that harmonizes the physical, emotional, mental, and spiritual dimensions of our being.

Love is the master harmony of the universe. The vibration of love is the crown of existence, the goal toward which we all are moving, the vibration that secretly animates this universe. To feel the profound bliss of love, its overpowering peace and profound depths in our daily life and relationships, is our highest fulfillment. This cannot be imposed but must emerge naturally. For this deep, inward vibration to be felt, consciousness must be still, coherent, and receptive. The soul, our psychic center, is spontaneously one with the vibration of Divine love. To come upon this state and express it in our lives is integral psychology's goal.

THE FURTHER REACHES OF
HUMAN TRANSFORMATION

Conventional psychology has given up on a human being realizing an enduring state of fulfillment, overflowing love, and abiding peace and happiness. At best, such things are fleeting, alternating with their opposites, and conventional wisdom maintains that most of life is a muddle somewhere in the middle. As long as human living is confined to the physical, emotional, and mental range of experience, this is perfectly true. The ordinary life of *samsara* is a ceaseless flux, oscillating between pleasure and pain, love and hate, and anxiety and safety. However, in the evolution of consciousness, there is a greater depth of being toward which humanity is moving.

Psychological transformation brings increasing *coherence*, while psychic transformation brings increasing *refinement*. Together they represent the next step in evolution—the growth of consciousness into its highest and widest fulfillment. With greater coherence and psychic refinement, new possibilities open up for relationship. We all long for connection and the fulfillment we experience in deep emotional resonance. The most complete and satisfying form of emotional resonance occurs in love. Love is the greatest attunement between two beings, and at its highest, it leads to union, the fullest resonance possible. This is not merger or loss of individuality; rather, it is an experience of joining together in the vibration of love, a state of utter completeness and relatedness. As the psychic transformation unfolds, relationship and resonance extend beyond other people to all of creation.

Transformation takes time. There is no getting around this hard fact of evolution. But if we invest ourselves, apply ourselves, and give ourselves a few decades for this important work, we will see a powerful, lasting change in ourselves, our relationships, and our world. The inner life is the only way out, the only satisfying answer to the problems of existence. Living from the inside out, refashioning our outer life from within by turning the powers of our inner being upon our surface nature, we can make our outer life a luminous expression of our deepest soul.

An evolutionary approach to health sees that

- there are depths to our subjectivity that far surpass previous views.
- the self is seen not just as a social construction or an error but as an evolutionary formation and expression of our deeper being.
- the developing soul has a unique evolutionary pathway, a purpose, a destiny, work to do, and lessons to learn. The growth of consciousness is the central fact of our life. "Good" is what facilitates the growth of our consciousness, and "bad" ("evil") is what impedes it.
- there is a source of self-existent bliss, light, love, peace, and power within us. It also is a source of wisdom and guidance that can be trusted completely. It is not merely socially constructed or culturally conditioned, although it is usually interpreted through our social and cultural conditioning. This deepest guidance can be trusted even when the mind does not know the reasons. For most of us, learning to discern the psychic center's quiet voice is a lifelong process (at least). Mistaking the mind's overconfident ideas, the heart's insistent impulsions and desires, and the body's habitual preferences for the soul's "still, quiet voice within" is an inevitable and a necessary part of our learning as the psychic center develops.
- states of cohesion or fragmentation become even more important, because they are seen to facilitate or block the deeper psychic guidance.
- beyond the psychological transformation that brings coherence to the self, the psychic transformation works to refine, purify, and psychicize the self so it becomes transparent, flexible, and responsive to the soul's light.
- the relational nature of the self expands to include our original and deepest relationship, to the Divine inwardly; from there it extends to all people and all creation outwardly.
- relationships that are of a psychic nature may be rare, but they are exceedingly precious. There is a role for all kinds of relationships, including those that are primarily mental, emotional, and physical, or some combination of each. As the psychic center comes forward, every relationship has its unique meaning.
- the inner heart becomes the center of embodied life.

- opening the heart is central to full living, so that the heart center can be a beacon in our life. When large portions of feeling life are unconscious and defensively repressed or disavowed, access to our psychic center is seriously impeded. Freeing up the heart and bringing it fully on-line is helpful in awakening the psychic flame.
- finding our authentic self is a guiding value in living. Although this does not in itself bring us to our psychic center, the authentic self is an important step along the way and a means of expressing our psychic center as our contact with it deepens.
- authentic relationships become a spiritual imperative. Creating our life from the inside out means reaching out, finding, and building the authentic relations that further our psychospiritual growth. Inauthentic relationships stifle and impede our unfolding, and as we grow, such relationships tend to shrivel and fall away, replaced by relationships and activities that reflect our true feelings and interests. Authentic self-expression is how the soul brings itself forth and participates in the world.
- love is the master harmony of life. To the degree that we can create and foster authentic, loving, and nourishing relationships, we approach a divine living. To the extent that negativity, toxic relationships, and harsh feelings characterize our relationships, we are living in hell. Learning to love authentically is a high priority (versus inauthentically living from images of a loving relationship and trying to force relationships into these images, a common form of spiritual bypassing that is epidemic and part of the legacy of Christian conditioning from which Western culture is still struggling to free itself).

In undergoing these two transformations, the self becomes more uniquely itself. It is not sameness or uniformity that evolution is heading toward but the opposite. Evolution creates ever-greater diversity, differentiation, and individuation. A soul-centered psychology sees that the highest function of psychological development and education is to cultivate individuality, developing one's authentic nature of body, heart, and mind while keeping the central focus of discovering one's psychic center. Each soul and self is distinct, an incomparable portion of Spirit. In entering ever more deeply into the depths of our unique psychic center, we experience our oneness with all—without losing our uniqueness. It is simultaneously union with all and a flowering of our individuality. In this we see how the Divine manifestation is an essential unity that expresses itself through an endless diversity of forms and selves. In diversity *is* unity, not dissolving one into the other but both existing in a rich harmony.

From this perspective, the task for non-Western cultures is to grow more in the direction of its members' individuality, freeing individuals' creative capacities for differentiation without losing the relational and social cohesion that is their source of strength. The task for Western cultures, on the other hand, is to grow more in the direction of relatedness and away from isolation and fragmentation, without losing the drive toward individuality that is the West's strength.

Greater relatedness and connection is the West's next evolutionary step. Yet it must be on a new, authentic basis, not on the old basis of obligation and meaningless family roles and ties, something outdated, outgrown, or dead or dying that deserves to be cast off as an impediment to a freer, more expansive life. Authentic connection must grow on a new psychological and spiritual basis of true relationship, genuine love and interest, real caring and respect, and truth in relating.

The central question is: How can this dual transformation be brought about? Which methods, practices, and discipline can we follow to awaken and bring forth increasing coherence and psychicization? That is the subject of the second half of this book.

Part 2

Integral Psychotherapy

Chapter 5

Psychotherapy As Behavior Change
Karma Yoga

Whatever a man's work and function in life, he can, if it is determined from
within or if he is allowed to make it a self-expression of his nature, turn it
into a means of growth and of a greater self-perfection.
—Sri Aurobindo, *Essays on the Gita*

The three powers of our human instrument—body, heart, and
mind—have produced in India three major paths to the Divine:

- The path of action in the world, or *karma* yoga
- The path of mindfulness and the mind, or *jnana* yoga
- The path of love and the heart, or *bhakti* yoga

Each traditional yoga uses the powers and capacities of one part of
our nature as a lever to lift us toward Spirit. In so doing, each yoga
develops splendidly one part of us but unfortunately neglects the other
two-thirds of our natural being.

Sri Aurobindo's integral yoga attempts to correct this one-sided
development with an integral growth of each part. It recognizes that
each person may favor or lead with one part, but that when carried to
the end, each path leads naturally to the others, culminating in a unity
of surrender, love, and knowledge.

It is the rich flowering of our whole being that we seek to develop.
Though in any particular lifetime we may emphasize one power more
than others, nevertheless it is an integral harmony that is our birthright

and evolutionary goal: body, heart, and mind raised to their full capacities, led by the psychic center through an increasingly psychicisized
and refined authentic self.

Individual differences have been problematic for the schools of psychotherapy, which often try to make one size fit all. But consciousness
is evolving along different pathways, and this must be considered in
inner development. The wisdom of Eastern psychology as embodied in
the three classical yogas recognizes that each individual has natural
routes for inner development—*karma* yoga, for action-oriented people
immersed in the world; *jnana* yoga, the path of the mind for contem-
plative natures; and *bhakti* yoga, the path of the heart for emotionally
attuned natures. The outer being or instrumental nature of body, heart,
and mind (the *koshas*) is being developed by the evolving soul in different ways. So, too, in psychotherapy—an integral psychotherapy must
allow for individual differences and be able to use what natural
strengths and abilities a client has to further the psychotherapeutic
process. One way of thinking about these differences lies through the
koshas and the classical yogas that spring from them.

Each gateway to the inner being is more accessible for certain
people than others, yet everyone has some way to make this inward
turning, even if it is only a first start. A first point of entry into the inner
world is through behavior. This pathway is open to everyone, even
those whose natural inclination is not to look within, for everyone acts.
Behaviorism has come upon a similar insight that behavior is universally available as a way to change. And, as we shall see, each pathway
eventually leads to, takes up, and includes the others when followed
along its natural direction, for in the end this is a path of wholeness and
integral evolution.

People generally enter psychotherapy in pain. Many clients are not
interested in why they are in pain, they just want it to go away and to
feel better. For such clients the natural starting point is a behavioral
approach. Psychotherapy of whatever persuasion finds that unskillful
behavior creates pain, and that feeling better comes by acting differently. This fundamental insight unites all schools of psychotherapy. The
differences between orientations consist only in how to best bring
about this change in behavior: behavior therapy uses outward means,
while depth therapy uses inner means.

In focusing on outwardly observable learning and behavior, behaviorism does not concern itself with deeper levels of consciousness, only

their visible, behavioral expressions. B. F. Skinner, the father of modern behaviorism, referred to behaviorism as a "black box" model of the psyche, meaning that behaviorism does not and should not speculate about the inner workings of consciousness but must stick to outwardly verifiable behavior. Only recently has behaviorism even admitted thinking as a valid area of study by classifying it as an internal behavior of talking to ourselves or "self-talk." Consequently, behavior therapy, cognitive therapy, and all of the various offshoots of cognitive-behavioral methods are concerned with getting clients to behave and think differently in order to reduce symptoms. The goal is behavior change, and any new awareness is an extraneous, though not unwelcome, accompaniment.

Feeling bad is feedback that indicates certain behavior does not meet our needs. Feeling better, in cognitive and behavioral therapies, comes by changing body, cognition, and behavior:

1. The body—for example, teaching relaxation techniques to reduce muscle tension, or teaching fuller, more relaxed diaphragmatic breathing; it also includes the use of physical means to directly change the brain's chemistry and to thus alter feeling states such as tranquilizers and anti-depressants.
2. Cognitions—challenging old thinking patterns and suggesting more rational thinking
3. Behavior—supporting the person in doing what is being avoided

Anxiety, stress, fear, and phobias are areas where cognitive-behavioral approaches have been shown to be most effective. Some types of depression and certain behavioral disorders such as bulimia and childhood conduct disorders also have shown some promising results when treated behaviorally. Although cognitive-behavioral methods are being used in other areas, these results have been more partial.

KARMA YOGA

Although all schools of psychotherapy deal with behavior, behaviorism and cognitive-behavioral therapies make most use of the vocabulary of behavior change. Similarly, while every world religion deals with the problem of action in the world, the Indian school of *karma* yoga specializes in this question. Karma yoga (*karma* means action, work, or works, though a more current translation might be behavior) is one of the three traditional Hindu yogas. The clearest and most influential articulation of karma yoga appears in the *Bhagavad Gita*, one of India's most revered sacred texts. The *Bhagavad Gita* is actually a small part of a much larger work, the *Mahabarata*, an epic Indian tale of a struggle between royal cousins over the rulership of an ancient Indian kingdom.

The essence of the story is a conflict between the forces of good and evil, where evil threatens to engulf the world, and the Divine forces must fight to restore the reign of the good. The forces of light are represented by five brothers, the Pandava princes, who lost their kingdom for a period of time in a rigged gambling game. The forces of evil and corruption are represented by the hundred sons of Kuru, who cheated the Pandava princes out of their kingdom. When the sons of Kuru refuse to give back the kingdom at the agreed time, the Pandavas must wage war to regain their rightful territory. But these two clans of the Pandavas and Kuru were raised together and have many relatives, teachers, and friends in common. War is a terrible prospect, because many family and close friends will be killed.

Krishna, an avatar or incarnation of God, is officially neutral in this dispute but lets Arjuna, the hero of the *Bhagavad Gita* and a great Pandava warrior, choose between having Krishna's army fight on his side or having Krishna as his charioteer. As the *Bhagavad Gita* begins, Arjuna has chosen Krishna as his charioteer and asks Krishna to drive his chariot to the very center of the battlefield between the two armies. Arjuna then looks out over both armies facing each other. As he surveys the scene, he sees sons, brothers, teachers, grandsons, uncles, and friends and realizes almost all of them will be killed in this great battle. At this dramatic moment, time freezes.

Arjuna is plunged into an existential crisis when he sees the devastation about to occur. He becomes overwhelmed with fear, grief, and the thought that even if he wins the battle, the slaughter of so many people he loves dearly will not be worth it. He throws down his bow and refuses to fight. He declares he wants to become a monk and to withdraw from the world.

The *Bhagavad Gita*, then, is a discourse by Krishna to Arjuna in which he enjoins Arjuna to stand up and fight, to stop avoiding his work as a warrior, and to lead the forces of justice in restoring righteousness to the world. But, counsels Krishna, fighting must not be done out of anger or fear but must flow from one's essential nature (*svabhava*) and as a spiritual practice. Krishna then takes Arjuna on a philosophical teaching in which action in the world becomes a means of liberation—karma yoga, or the yoga of action. In karma yoga, all of our activities are to be done as a form of worship, in a spirit of surrender to the Divine and openness to Divine guidance. By the end of the *Gita* Arjuna picks up his bow and joins the battle, which is finally won by the Pandavas at a great cost to both sides as the *Mahabarata* continues.

Each of us, of course, is Arjuna on the battlefield of life—anxious, scared, and overwhelmed at the existential realities of loss and death, confused about what to do, and tempted to withdraw and avoid the stresses of the world. In the face of Arjuna's refusal to fight, Krishna, as the divine teacher, does what any good behavior therapist would do— he works with Arjuna to change his behavior. Krishna works on two levels: changing Arjuna's outward phobic behavior of avoiding battle, and changing Arjuna's inward behavior, his thinking, by changing his cognitive framework. Arjuna's fear is apparent in his graphic description of his physical symptoms. Arjuna says:

My limbs sink down
And my mouth dries up
And my body trembles
And my hair stands on end. (Sargeant, 1984, I, 29)

Krishna initially responds rather unempathically and even shamingly in his initial attempt to get Arjuna to change his behavior:

Whence this timidity of thine,
Come to thee in time of danger,
Not acceptable in an Aryan, not leading to heaven
Causing disgrace, Arjuna?
Do not become a coward . . .
This, in thee, is not suitable.
Abandoning base faintheartedness,
Stand up! Scorcher of the foe. (Sargeant, 1984, II, 2–3)

Cognitive-behavior therapy works most effectively with phobias and fears of various kinds. Phobic behavior maintains itself by reinforcing the fear every time the feared object is avoided. The essential therapeutic strategy for eliminating phobic behavior is to confront what is avoided. Just as Arjuna's initial fear on the battlefield caused him to recoil and avoid behaving as a warrior, Krishna works to change his thinking patterns and behavior, to face the enemy and engage the battle, to act according to his nature rather than out of fear. Thus the *Gita* recommends exposure to what is feared—the great behavioral prescription, for what decades of psychological research into fear have discovered is that *exposure heals fear.*

However, it should be noted that not just any kind of exposure is healing, for exposure accompanied by fear and distress can simply reinforce fear. It must be a safe and controlled exposure, done with a relatively relaxed body and calm mind. Here the *Gita* encompasses the truth of controlled exposure and surpasses it when Krishna tells Arjuna that his action is not to be done in an agitated state or in anger but must be done from a state of deep peace and equality. This peace and equality come out of the inner spirit, and it is from these depths that action must ultimately spring.

Cognitive-behavioral therapy produces a reduced version of this by teaching relaxation strategies and changing catastrophic, rigid thinking patterns, then proceeding with controlled exposure to the feared situation. For example, in working with a man who has a bridge phobia, a behavior therapist may teach him how to relax his muscles and to breathe from his belly as he relaxes. Drugs also may be prescribed for relaxation. The therapist challenges the man's catastrophic thinking and gets him to reevaluate more realistically the actual danger of bridges. Then the therapist works with the man to gradually walk toward a bridge. As the man's anxiety increases, the man would be instructed to stop or back up a few steps, to relax and calm down before proceeding. Then the therapist would encourage him to approach the bridge again. As the man's anxiety builds, the therapist counsels him to stop and relax. This stop-start pattern continues until gradually the man is standing in the middle of the bridge. In surrendering illogical to logical cognitions, in surrendering contracted muscles for relaxation, and in surrendering avoidance of bridges to exposure to other bridges, the man's bridge phobia is resolved, and he is able to act differently.

Depression is the other major symptom for which cognitive-behavioral therapy can be effective. Arjuna speaks to Krishna not only of anxiety and fear, he also speaks of overwhelming grief and depression from the death of so many loved ones. With "this sorrow of mine which dries up the senses," Arjuna declares that he is better off being killed himself than killing others, as the *Gita's* first chapter, "The Despondency of Arjuna," ends by Arjuna

> Throwing down both bow and arrow,
> With a heart overcome by sorrow. (Sargeant, 1984, I, 47)

Like a master cognitive-behavioral therapist, Krishna works first to change Arjuna's thinking by reframing this battle and explaining that there is nothing to grieve. No one really dies, for the true soul is immortal. All that dies is the body, for that which is born must die. What is there to mourn in this natural event?

> Truly there was never a time when I was not,
> Nor thou, nor these lords of men;
> And neither will there be a time when we shall cease to be; . . .
> No one is able to accomplish
> The destruction of this imperishable (the atman.)
> Neither is this (atman) born nor does it die at any time,
> Nor, having been, will it again come not to be.
> Birthless, eternal, perpetual, primeval,
> It is not slain when the body is slain . . .
> As, after casting away worn out garments,
> A man later takes new ones,
> So, after casting away worn out bodies,
> The atman encounters other, new ones . . .
> For the born, death is certain;
> For the dead there is certainly birth.
> Therefore, for this, inevitable in consequence,
> Thou shouldst not mourn. (Sargeant, 1984, II, 12, 22, 27)

Arjuna is heartened by Krishna's words. But though Krishna's reframing helps reduce his depressive feelings, Arjuna seeks more than this. Just as a cognitive-behavioral approach to anxiety and depression oftentimes works, at other times it is not enough. Directly changing behavior and cognitions is an important dimension in psychotherapy. It is a surface approach that produces a surface change in behavior, thinking, and feeling. For certain clients it is sufficient to reduce symptoms to a tolerable level, for this is all many clients are concerned with, so behaviorism and drugs may be enough. Indeed, given the current evolutionary level of humanity, it is no wonder that behaviorism and drugs are such popular methods of treatment, for there has not yet entered into the general population the power of a deeper and more inward living. Additionally, given the limitations of many life circumstances, for example, a depressed elderly client whose faculties are failing, and who has neither the time nor resources for depth psychotherapy, drugs and behavior therapy may be the best that can be reasonably expected. But a cognitive-behavioral strategy is only a first approach to changing behavior.

While drugs and cognitive-behavioral therapies have their place, human psychology is more complex than these approaches comprehend. For many other people, behavior therapy and drugs are ineffective or achieve only temporary results. Clients often sense that there is much more to their issues than a simple Band-Aid can remedy. The schools of depth psychotherapy seek to understand these larger domains of the human psyche. They begin to lay their hands on the deeper levers of human behavior to effect change.

Like many clients, Arjuna is not satisfied merely with a behavioral prescription or a cognitive reorientation. He prods Krishna to go farther to unlock the secret of right action. And the teaching of the *Gita* is more profound than just getting Arjuna to act differently. By the end of the *Gita* Arjuna not only behaves differently but acts from a different consciousness. Action in the world (behavior) as a field for the growth of consciousness is the *Gita's* greater message.

AN INTEGRATING PRINCIPLE FOR EAST AND WEST

Eastern psychology is a ringing refutation of postmodernism's denial of deeper realities. The unanimous testimony of Eastern psychology is that there is indeed a core being beyond our frontal ego, if only we have the eyes to see it. This inner being is something to which the Western depth psychologies have been intuitively pointing, but only vaguely and imprecisely. Further, as we enlarge our view of psychology, we see that this essential being includes and surpasses the frontal physical-emotional-mental self.

Integral psychology draws on the yogic understanding of essential being or uniqueness as a unifying principle of wholeness. The Sanskrit word *svabhava* (pronounced *sva - bha' - va*) means our essential nature or uniqueness, and it can be translated in many ways, including intrinsic self, inherent nature, or self-being. This essential nature is inherent in our spiritual being. As it develops over many lives, the influence of the spiritual nature increases, so that more and more of the frontal self follows one's *svabhava*. What Western psychology studies as the *authentic self* is but an expression of the inner, essential uniqueness that Indian psychology studies as the *soul* or *psychic center*.

Indian spirituality has declared for thousands of years that with a spiritual aspiration, we can follow our authentic nature to a higher, spiritual fulfillment. Following our *svabhava* leads to a path of self-realization (*svadharma*) or action that follows the authentic development of the self. In India's most revered sacred text, the *Bhagavad Gita*, Krishna states that one's intrinsic nature can lead to the highest spiritual liberation:

> By worshipping with his own proper action (*svadharma*)
> Him from Whom beings have their origin,
> Him by Whom all this universe is pervaded,
> A person finds perfection.
> Better one's own innate action (*svadharma*), though imperfect,
> Than the innate action of another well performed.
> One should not abandon one's inborn action
> Even though it be deficient,
> Indeed, all undertakings are enveloped in deficiency
> As fire is in smoke. (Sargeant, 1984, XVIII 46–48)

Krishna, who like Christ or Buddha is seen as a divine teacher, here states a central teaching of the *Gita*. Following one's own essential nature leads to liberation. Following another's path is dangerous for the soul (III 35) and blocks our inner growth, for it is external and imposed upon our genuine inner being. Even if we are more outwardly successful at something foreign to us, or even if our own path seems defective, we must realize that all human work is deficient to some extent. That should not make us abandon our own unique path and gifts. Indeed, through meditation and inner discipline, we can align our life and actions with our essential nature (*svabhava*) and reach a supreme spiritual perfection.

This is very much in accord with the teachings of modern psychology. Although Western psychology has not yet fully understood the nature of our essential being, it points toward an authentic self through which we find ourselves and fulfillment. Western psychology has not comprehended the deeper, spiritual nature of our essential being, but it does recognize the importance of honoring our unique nature. Here, in a nutshell, is the reason what psychology calls self-actualization feels so good and so right, for in a larger, more integral view, self-actualization is part of a larger process of spiritual unfolding. Self-actualization touches into the deeper essential spiritual being without fully recognizing it.

The quest for wholeness is a search for the full integrality of our being—body, heart, mind, and spirit. On the psychological level, this is a search for the authentic self, an integrated, cohesive self that is an expression of our true nature. Psychological healing and growth are important steps toward this but are not sufficient, for full integrality is rooted in spirit, and only as the quest for wholeness comes to include the deeper spiritual aspiration does it move toward fulfillment.

DEPTH PSYCHOTHERAPY AND BEHAVIOR CHANGE

Using action and behavior as a way to expand awareness is another way to approach behavior change. Depth psychotherapy seeks to change behavior through deepening awareness. Limited consciousness results in limited behaviors that produce pain. Expanding consciousness yields expanded behavioral possibilities. From this greater freedom flows more skillful and more rewarding behavior. Behavior changes with greater consciousness.

Action and behavior run on a continuum from more subtle behaviors such as talking and thinking to more outwardly dramatic expressions such as hitting or yelling. We cannot help but act, as Krishna points out:

> Indeed, no one, even in the twinkling of an eye,
> Ever exists without performing action . . .

And even the mere maintenance of thy body
Could not be accomplished without action. (Sargeant, 1984, III,
5,8)

While action-oriented therapies often disparage verbalization as
"just talk," it is through the action of talking that most people interact
and spend most of their interpersonal lives. And it is through the action
of thinking that we make sense of the world and orient our lives. While
most of the psychotherapy field enters the psyche through talking, a
number of depth psychotherapies, such as gestalt, bioenergetics, drama
therapy, and psychodrama, use more expressive behaviors and action.
Their strategy is to use such techniques as role-playing, behavioral
experiments, voice exercises, exaggerating or suppressing behaviors,
contracting and relaxing muscles, breathwork, hitting pillows, and
trying on new behaviors to enhance awareness in the movement toward
behavior change.

For example, with most therapists a woman client with relationship
issues would spend the hour talking about her feelings and relationships. Depending upon the orientation of the therapist, she would be
encouraged to explore her deeper feelings, their childhood roots, and
how her current patterns may be a replay of earlier family relationships,
as well as how these patterns also show up in her relationship with her
therapist and other people in her current life. An action-oriented therapist might suggest that she role-play her husband, her father, her
mother, and other significant relationships in order to bring greater
awareness to her feelings. Whether a therapist uses words or action
techniques, the underlying assumption is that we discover ourselves
through our actions, our words, and our behavior.

When time freezes at the beginning of the *Gita*, a sacred space is
created in which only Arjuna and Krishna seem to exist. About two-
thirds of the way through their dialogue, Krishna provides Arjuna with
a profound experience of Krishna as the all-pervading godhead. Its
effect upon Arjuna is powerfully mind-boggling and humbling, and it
shakes Arjuna to the core. An astonished Arjuna sees Krishna in a new
light, and from that point on he takes his discourse far more seriously.
In a similar way, psychotherapy must be a profound and an intense
experience if it is to be healing and growth inspiring.

Whatever behavioral pathway is used, whether words or actions, it
must not remain "just talking" or even "just hitting or just yelling," even

though these may be intense or lead to some kind of discharge. It must lead to inner deepening. It is the deepening of experience that engages the client on the inner journey. Psychotherapy is the creation of a sacred space where inner depths can be plumbed. The boundaries that form the psychotherapeutic container for psychotherapy, such as a consistent time frame, space, fee, confidentiality, and so on, make for a safe space in which to open and explore new depths.

Expecting specific, immediate results impedes the exploration of inner depths. Psychotherapy is a *process*, and it is by attending to the client's inner process that inner deepening occurs. The *Gita's* teaching is very much in accord with psychotherapy in this regard, for it also counsels attending to process rather than focusing upon results. This comes by offering the results of all actions to God, letting go of the fruits of action, and focusing upon the action itself. This allows consciousness to deepen by bringing peace and equality into everyday acts. As Krishna says:

> Thy jurisdiction is in action alone;
> Never in its fruits at any time.
> Never should the fruits of action be thy motive. (Sargeant, 1984, II, 47)

The unfolding of the self in psychotherapy always occurs in surprising and unexpected ways. It does not always proceed along the stages according to a particular school's map. As all therapists learn but soon forget, such maps are helpful but must be held lightly, otherwise there is the danger of missing the territory by fixating on the map.

FROM UNSKILLFUL BEHAVIOR
TO SKILLFUL BEHAVIOR

"Yoga is skill in actions," Krishna tells Arjuna in the *Bhagavad Gita*. A more modern rendering might be, "Yoga is skillful behavior." From one perspective, neurosis consists of unskillful behavior. Psychological health is skillful behavior.

Karma yoga aims at skillful behavior through surrender: surrendering our desires and ego-based living to the Divine, to allow our spiritual nature to emerge and guide our life. Psychotherapy also can be seen as a process of surrender: surrender to our deeper self, surrendering neurotic over-control so that our authentic nature may emerge and guide our life.

When we act from the false self, we create needless pain for ourselves, for we are acting out of the original coping strategy we developed in our family of origin. This served us at the time. It shielded us from our pain and allowed us to cope with the wounded psyches of our mother, father, and other family members. It was, at the time, a creative adaptation to difficult circumstances. The problem is that the self becomes fixated in a given coping pattern. The self develops only along certain lines that are reinforced in the original system, deficits in the self's structure are inevitably created, and false, defensive structures compensate for these gaps. Because the self's development gets arrested, the self becomes tied into acting in repetitive ways, which Freud called the repetition compulsion. The self looks for love in the same ways that it looked for love in the original family, for example, by being attracted to men or women who are unavailable in similar ways as father or mother was. The self is trying to work out the original wounding, trying to complete the unfinished gestalt from childhood, but unfortunately it keeps recreating the scenario in ways that keep it incomplete, and it reinforces the old patterns. This unskillful behavior creates unnecessary pain.

Depth psychotherapy changes this by changing one's consciousness. By healing old wounds, filling in the deficits in the self's structure, exploring behavioral patterns in relationships, and freeing up the static object relations matrix that perpetuates repetitive patterns, new behavioral possibilities open up. Depth psychotherapy proceeds little by little in "peeling the onion" of the psyche. As defenses erode, deeper feelings emerge, which in turn will give way to new layers of defenses that need further working through. Gradually the early wounds and roots of the psyche are exposed, cleansed, and healed. This process alters the balance of forces in the psyche. As the inner forces of the psyche shift, there is a resulting shift in behavior. The goal of all depth psychotherapy is to act from a deeper source, increasingly from the authentic self.

Acting from our deeper, authentic nature allows us to act more skillfully, for we then are in full possession of our powers, no longer hampered by having much of our feeling, sensing, and thinking self repressed and unavailable. Neurosis is like operating with impaired vision and hearing and without the use of an arm and a leg. Of course, neurotic behavior is unskillful, for the self is operating at only partial capacity. But in acting from our authentic depths, we more skillfully navigate our life's course and are able to find relationships that truly nourish us rather than perpetually frustrate us and to find our true calling, a form of creative work that integrates our ambitions, skills, and ideals. Freud once defined the cure of neurosis as "the ability to love and to work," but the profundity of his statement is easily missed. Love and work are the two major dimensions of embodied life. Pain results when either sphere is frustrated.

The need for deep, intimate, vulnerable, and loving relationships is by now fairly well known. But the importance for a creative work that employs the self's full capacities is often overlooked. Alienation from work is so widespread that it is taken for granted. Having to work is often seen as a burden, one of life's necessary hardships. Yet work is our primary way of engaging the world. Finding true work, and having this develop and mature over one's lifespan, brings an incomparable depth of fulfillment.

The paramount significance of authentic work is one of the *Gita's* strongest messages. "By works the worlds are created," say Krishna, "Without works the world would fall into ruin." Following our true nature (*swadharma*) leads us to our proper work and, further, can become a means of spiritual development.

What the *Gita* teaches is that developing the capacities we have leads to right livelihood and our true direction in life, the means by which our deeper self (*svabhava*) can manifest, and further, that such action can lead to spiritual liberation. Without using the language of psychology, the *Gita* provides the spiritual basis for self-actualization.

In karma yoga what is paramount is the consciousness with which we work. Work that flows from our essential, authentic nature (*svabhava*) engages the full self—our gifts and capacities. This kind of engagement produces a state of "flow" (Csikszentmihalyi, 1990, 1997), a state where our consciousness is in harmony with its own nature and action is a free outflowing of our being. Such work is simultaneously the most fulfilling and the most growth enhancing for our evolving consciousness. *Work is a field for the growth of consciousness*—this is the whole pith and sense of the *Bhagavad Gita*, and it is a psychological and a spiritual fulfillment.

If the growth of consciousness is the secret meaning of life on earth and the central principle of the self, then whatever aids our growth may be broadly defined as "good," even though it may be unpleasant, and whatever retards our growth can be seen as "bad" or evil, even though pleasant. Karma (action, behavior, activity, work) is the means for our unfolding in the world. Work, as our primary way of engaging the world, then assumes the utmost importance. Alienating work that does not make use of our true capacities may be regarded as toxic to the self or bad. Work that is in alignment with our self and provides a rich environment for self-unfolding and self-expression is to be highly valued.

The dream of making enough money to retire and stop working reflects a person's alienation from work. When work is a creative engagement of the self's capacities, work is a joy and fulfillment. *Not* working is then the tragedy, along with the fragmentation and ensuing withdrawal into distractions, pleasure, or numbing entertainment.

Krishna enjoins Arjuna to perform his true work as a warrior, and it is clear to all that this is his sacred duty. In a simpler world, where family and society determined much of a person's work and relationships, such choices were more limited. Sri Aurobindo, in line with other important philosophical thinkers who came after him, such as Jean Gebser and Teilhard de Chardin, saw society evolve as individual consciousness evolved. He posited an evolutionary development in society from earlier forms that are typal and conventional, where a person's place in the world is entirely regulated by outer circumstances, such as family and society, as was the case in medieval Europe and India. As evolution proceeds, these give way to societies that are more rational, individualistic, and subjective, that offer and demand more individual choice, such as the increasingly complex and specialized modern world. As individuals evolve, they become more complex and differentiated and, as a consequence, society becomes more complex and differentiated. For the growing soul, an increasing self-awareness accompanies this evolutionary development, and earlier, more primitive forms of society become constraining, because they limit the freedom and growth that come with choice.

However, the increasing freedom and choice that accompany evolution's greater "complexification," as De Chardin termed it, cannot be navigated merely with an increasingly complex mind but will require deeper self-awareness. It is in this evolutionary context of a more individualistic and subjective world that psychotherapy arises. Itself a product of life's increasing complexification, psychotherapy increases self-awareness and individuation. In today's complicated world, the discovery of meaningful work that engages our total self—our capacities, ambitions, ideals—demands a degree of self-awareness that neurosis often blocks. Depth therapy works to melt these blocks to self-awareness so our true calling becomes clear.

OPENING AND SURRENDER

The teaching of the *Gita* is that our action (behavior) can be a path to spiritual realization. The *Gita* prescribes opening and surrender: opening to the Divine and the surrender of our will to the Divine will, surrender of our motivation (desires) to the aspiration for the Divine, surrender of ego to Self or self to spirit, surrender of ego-centered activity to Divine service, surrender of self-determination and mental guidance to a higher, Divine leading. Depth psychotherapy utilizes the same principles of opening and surrender in its work with the frontal self. Psychotherapy involves opening to the inner depths of the psyche and progressively surrendering to its wiser guidance. It is a surrender of the false self to the authentic self, a surrender of fear and defenses to faith in the authentic self's abilities, a surrender of ego control to organismic wisdom.

However, this psychological transformation does not happen overnight. It is a progressive process of healing, growth, and slow transformation. First there is a turning within to feel and sense deeper realms of our being. Inevitably, inner layers of shielding are encountered that prevent further deepening, and this takes time to work through. In opening to the deeper layers of the psyche, painful though they may be, there is a sense of coming home, coming back to ourselves, of feeling more solid, more substantial, more real than ever before. As the false self gives way, the true self begins to come forth. We discover more fully how we truly feel, what we truly need in our relationships versus what we thought we needed, where our interests and talents lie, and what our true work is. In short, our authentic, essential self or intrinsic nature (*svabhava*) is discovered. The *Gita* declares that following our *svabhava* as a spiritual practice leads to our spiritual ground.

In the language of integral psychology, in opening and surrendering to our authentic self we come into greater alignment with our evolving soul and essential nature. Our aspiration for the true consciousness, for wholeness, becomes a passage toward our spiritual nature, self-actualization leading to Self-realization. It becomes a way to discover our spiritual being. This aspiration is not the ego's desire but the soul's need. Tuning into this inherent aspiration lights a fire in the heart that begins to change the course of our life and guide us in the right direction.

What is necessary in this deepening aspiration is faith, a word that has been corrupted in the West by its long association with mere belief. But as the Christian mystics testify and the *Gita* confirms, faith goes far beyond belief. The *Gita* even goes so far as to say:

> Man is made of faith.
> Whatever faith he has, thus he is. (Sargeant, 1984, XVII, 3)

The power of human consciousness is such that it manifests what it focuses on. If a man thinks of himself as worthless, then his ensuing depression soon confirms this judgment. Cognitive therapy attempts to exchange this man's faith in his worthlessness for a thinking and feeling pattern that honors his value so the depression will lift. All psychotherapy proceeds on faith in our greater possibilities.

> Faith does not depend upon experience; it is something that is there before experience. When one starts the yoga, it is not usually on the strength of experience, but on the strength of faith. It is so not only in yoga and the spiritual life, but in ordinary life also. All men of action, discoverers, inventors, creators of knowledge proceed by faith and, until the proof is made or the thing done, they go on in spite of disappointment, failure, disproof, denial because of something in them that tells them that this is the truth, the thing that must be followed and done. Ramakrishna even went so far as to say, when asked whether blind faith was not wrong, that blind faith was the only kind to have, for faith is either blind or it is not faith but something else—reasoned inference, proved conviction or ascertained knowledge.
> Faith is the soul's witness to something not yet manifested, achieved or realized, but which yet the Knower within us, even in the absence of all indications, feels to be true or supremely worth following or achieving. (Aurobindo, 1971a, p. 572)

During the first period of the soul's growth, faith in spirit is weak and faith in sensory reality and all things physical predominates, creating a materialistic life lived mainly on the surface. As the evolving soul matures, faith in spirit grows stronger, and inner psychological and spiritual realities emerge more clearly. As faith in the soul's aspiration for wholeness develops, this aspiration proves itself in the end by transforming utterly the entire experience of living. Depending upon the vision and faith of a client, psychotherapy leads to very different outcomes. For some clients, psychotherapy will stay limited to the small field of behavior change. For others, behavior will be a stepping-stone to inner deepening. Behavior as a way to deepen consciousness, to discover and act from the authentic self can, the *Gita* teaches, proceed even further to the discovery of the inner spirit.

One reason for the *Gita's* preeminent place in India's sacred literature is its widely embracing vision of the Divine as both Personal and Impersonal, along with its acceptance of different spiritual paths. Depending upon one's nature, one can travel the path of action in the world (karma yoga), the path of the mind or mindfulness (jnana yoga), or the path of the heart or devotion (bhakti yoga.) The *Gita* concedes that the impersonal path of the atman or Buddha-nature is steep, strenuous, and inaccessible to all but a very few.

> The exertion of those whose minds
> Are fixed on the Unmanifest is greater;
> The goal of the Unmanifest is attained
> With difficulty by embodied beings. (Sargeant, 1984, XII, 5)

The easier and more natural path for the great majority lies through the heart. Krishna holds a revered place in Indian tradition as the object of devotion in many of the bhakti schools of Vedanta, and this is reflected in the *Gita's* preference for the path of the heart. The heart is the seat of the immanent Divine, as the *Gita* makes clear in this reference to the soul, located deep within the heart center.

> The Lord abides in the heart
> Of all beings, Arjuna. (Sargeant, 1984, XVIII, 61)

Karma yoga is a surrender of our ego to the Divine. Psychotherapy is a surrender of our irrational beliefs and behaviors to more rational beliefs and behaviors; more deeply, it is a surrender of our limited, fear-based behavior patterns to a greater range of risk taking and reaching out; deeper still, it is a surrender of our neurotic, false self to our authentic self. Finally, integral psychotherapy encompasses these and includes a surrender of our outer living and surface self to our inner being and psychic center.

DOING PSYCHOTHERAPY AS KARMA YOGA

Being a psychotherapist also becomes a practice of *karma* yoga. It becomes a process of dedication and offering work to the Divine, of opening to inner guidance, and the (very difficult) process of letting go of the fruit of the reward. The first step is consecration, or dedicating one's life to the Divine, which not only karma yoga but every spiritual tradition advocates.

In psychotherapy consecration is dedicating oneself to "becoming a pro" as Bugental (1978) puts it. This means dedication to working on ourselves psychologically, in our own therapy and lives, as well as developing a commitment to our professional growth as lifelong learners. The learnings of psychotherapy are profoundly life changing, affecting relationships and who we relate to, how deeply and intimately we can go in our relationships, and our relationship to ourselves, our feelings, our body, and our dreams. Each therapist changes in different ways through his or her own inner work, and psychological growth is a process without end.

Consecrating ourselves to becoming a professional is the first level; the second is consecrating ourselves to the Divine. This means concentrating all of our energies on this one aspiration, which we cannot do—at least the surface self cannot do it, since it runs in so many other directions. In integral yoga and integral psychotherapy, this dilemma is resolved by seeing the need for a central, harmonizing focus, an integrating center around which to organize our life. This central organizing principle is the psychic center. The aspiration for awakening becomes paramount in becoming an integral psychotherapist.

A second aspect of therapy as karma yoga is surrender. Depth psychotherapy involves a progressive surrender to our deeper, authentic self. Integral yoga psychotherapy carries this a step farther in surrendering our entire being to the Divine. Here again, what the frontal self cannot do, the psychic center can. We can give all of ourselves to the Divine and surrender our desire for the fruit of the reward to whatever result the Divine deems best.

Giving up our attachment to the reward and focusing on the work itself is probably the best advice that can be given to a psychotherapist (or anyone, for that matter). Yet there is nothing harder to do, for one of the most central motives for human beings is to feel competent. Self-esteem is directly linked to competence. We do something well and feel good about ourselves; we do something poorly and feel bad about ourselves. Some personality theorists maintain that competence is the basis for all of personality development (see, e.g., Basch, 1988). For the therapist, this is a real dilemma, since feeling effective is essential to feeling good about ourselves. For example, we want our clients to get better, to improve, to feel better, and to move on in their lives, partly because we compassionately want them to get better and partly because we want to feel competent and good about ourselves. When clients do poorly or therapy fails, the self-esteem of the therapist suffers, and anguish results. Letting go of outcome is *very* difficult to do.

One way of resolving this is to differentiate reward as feedback about process versus reward as the goal. In seeing the reward (clients getting better) as feedback, the focus is still on the process—receiving necessary information about whether the work is moving in the right direction or not. If the client is dissatisfied with the therapy, then this is essential feedback. Perhaps something is off or a transference disruption is occurring that needs attention. Either way, it is a way of focusing on the process. This is quite different from focusing on the reward as a goal, for instance, a business that focuses just on the bottom line and pegs self-worth to net worth.

Opening to the Divine for guidance, for healing, and for spirit's transformational energies is another aspect of psychotherapy as karma yoga. Opening to the Divine for guidance and intuition can be tricky, because this can be a cover for opening to our own unconscious—our needs for power, for love, for looking smart, for admiration—or to subtle energies and beings from the intermediate plane. All we open to may not be the Divine. The psychological literature is full of warnings about the dangers of blindly following our own "intuition" and clinical hunches, since these often are rationales for indulging our own countertransference feelings or acting out impulses that are not in the best interests of the client. Similarly, the spiritual literature is full of warnings about opening the dangers of blindly following whatever lesser lights or inner forces we find inside, for these may not all be of the highest origin—they may even be hostile or anti-Divine forces. Here again it is the discrimination provided by the psychic center that is crucial in steering clear of these dangers.

Finally, the concept of *svabhava* is important. Is being a psychotherapist part of our *svabhava* or essential nature? Is it right livelihood and an authentic expression of our true self? If so, what is our *svadharma*, or our unique style of psychotherapy? Which kind of orientation, which techniques, and which types of clients do we work best with? Discovering what psychological methods we resonate with most fully, and the parts of our being that we are developing in this lifetime, reflects which schools of therapy we gravitate toward. In honoring our *svabhava* and individual path of development, this leads us toward our psychic center. As the psychic center emerges, as we consciously make the Divine more central in our lives and work, our outer practice of psychotherapy becomes a means for opening to spirit.

Psychotherapy becomes a means of working on ourselves as we make our work an offering to the Divine. Psychotherapy is service to the Divine that allows us to bring forth into our outer nature the inner realizations. In the path of transformation, inner realization is not enough; only a change of our entire outer being is complete, therefore, karma yoga is an essential dimension of an integral working.

CONCLUSION

In this enlarged vision of psychotherapy as a form of karma yoga, the goal includes behavior change and increased coherence as the authentic self comes on-line and defensive structures of the false self dissipate; but it goes beyond these conventional goals to identify the source of the authentic self as the evolving soul or psychic center, whose influence, power, and consciousness increasingly become the guiding light and center of consciousness. Greater psychicization is integral psychology's goal, accompanied by the self's greater coherence. This integrates East and West in an enlarged vision of karma yoga, synthesizing the East's deeper maps and methods with the West's more precise understanding of the ego and the unconscious for an integral working.

Besides karma yoga, two other key paths have evolved for finding spirit. The path of the mind (jnana yoga) uses mindfulness and discrimination to discover atman or Buddha-nature. The path of the heart (bhakti yoga) uses devotion, love, surrender, bhakti, and aspiration to discover the psychic center or true soul. These two pathways to the inner depths, mindfulness and heartfulness, have profound implications for psychotherapy, and an integrally comprehensive psychotherapy incorporates both.

Chapter 6

Psychotherapy As Mindfulness Practice
Jnana Yoga

> Consciousness is a fundamental thing, the fundamental thing in existence—it is the energy, the motion, the movement of consciousness that creates the universe and all that is in it—not only the macrocosm but the microcosm is nothing but consciousness arranging itself.
> —Sri Aurobindo, *Letters on Yoga*

Beginning in India with Buddha about 600 B.C.E., together with Lao-Tzu in China, Shankara in India, and culminating with modern teachers of the Impersonal Divine, such as Krishnamurti and Ramana Maharshi, the East has produced a steady stream of teachers of mindfulness as a path to realization. Buddhism, Taoism, and *kevala advaita* Vedanta all reveal the Spirit as an infinite, impersonal consciousness, the atman that is Brahman and the all-pervading ground from which all arises. The path to atman (or Buddha-nature) is called *jnana* yoga, which uses mindfulness or the mind's discrimination to sift through the mind's illusions and discover the foundation of consciousness.

The path of mindfulness is the path of the eternal Now. All that exists is this present moment—right here, right now. But the ego lives in the past and future, spinning out fantasies and inhabiting a kind of virtual reality that is more akin to dreaming or being half asleep. Because of gross desires for things, people, sensory pleasure, and avoidance of pain, consciousness becomes dull, tied to a fixed groove of sleepwalking. The spiritual practice of mindfulness penetrates this habitual stream of reactions and begins the process of awakening.

111

Many varieties of witness consciousness or mindfulness practice have been developed by different traditions. Tibetan Buddhism refers to mindfulness, in Theravada Buddhism it is called bare attention or *vipassana*, and in Zen Buddhism it is known as *zazen*. Krishnamurti's non-method of "choiceless awareness" is a contemporary rendering of this ancient Buddhist practice into a more modern vocabulary. Similarly, Gurdjieff's "self-remembering" is yet another variant. In India's Samkya tradition, as well as in Sri Aurobindo's integral yoga, it appears as the process of detaching the observer from the nature (*prakriti*), a standing back from the contents of consciousness to discover a silent witness within. In the *kevala advaita* tradition, the mind's discriminative awareness discerns the real and eternal atman from all that is noneternal and illusory. Nisargadatta Maharaj's searching for who seeks and Ramana Maharshi's method of self-inquiry and progressive disidentification from body, heart, and mind also are contemporary versions of this practice.

The many varieties of mindfulness practice that have evolved share some central characteristics. Essentially, mindfulness is a process of paying attention to whatever arises in consciousness, bringing full awareness to our experience, awareness of thoughts, feelings, and sensations rather than being carried away mindlessly by their flow. Mindfulness practice in some Buddhist traditions begins by focusing on the breath—paying careful attention to the many subtle sensations of breathing in and out. This is a first stage of mindfulness, and when concentration increases and attention can witness the depths of physical sensations of breathing, the practice then expands to whatever feelings, thoughts, and fantasies arise in consciousness. There is no directive other than to observe whatever arises and passes away, like watching a cloud pass in the sky, observing without judgment, condemnation, or justification. Observing in this way becomes an inquiry into the self, and insight develops that reveals the nature of mind.

Through observation and awareness, the mind's habitual activity settles down. As it becomes still, the mind becomes like a polished mirror that reflects back whatever it sees with pristine clarity. At some point, awareness expands to see how the ego is itself a series of thoughts and images put together moment to moment out of desire and memory. In penetrating the spaces between these images, we enter a vast and an impersonal emptiness that shows our fundamental identity to be pure consciousness rather than the *contents* of consciousness with which we usually identify (i.e., bodily sensations, feelings, impulses, thoughts, and images). This pure consciousness is none other than the atman that is Brahman, one without a second.

From the negative side, called *Nirguna* Brahman, this is a void, a no-thing-ness, an emptiness beyond all forms. Forms are revealed to be ultimately empty, and this emptiness is seen to be the support of all forms ("Form is emptiness, emptiness is form," as the famous Buddhist sutra proclaims). It is the Tao, the impersonal movement beyond all words. It is a void that is entirely empty and therefore infinitely full of everything.

From the positive side, called *Saguna* Brahman, this is a state of pure, blissful Being, a Self existence beyond ego, a source of identity containing all wisdom, eternally at rest, a silence that supports every-thing, an Impersonal witness that sees all equally in a profound silence, the source and goal of all. The Sanskrit terms *sat, chit,* and *ananda* are the three positive descriptors of Brahman—existence, consciousness, and bliss. Brahman is an infinitely blissful, conscious existence out of which everything comes.

The *jnana* yoga path to this consists of various types of mindful-ness practice designed to still the mind and end all identification with one's outer body, heart, and mind. When the mind slows down and becomes silent, mindful discrimination can penetrate the ego's thoughts to find the underlying reality of pure consciousness.

MINDFULNESS AND PSYCHOTHERAPY

Applying mindfulness to psychotherapy frames the therapeutic process in terms of consciousness. This harkens back to Freud's view of the goal of therapy—*to make the unconscious conscious*—but goes well beyond his ideas about what the unconscious is and what the possibilities are for full consciousness. Unconscious defenses result in fixation and develop-mental arrest. Psychotherapy brings attention to these avoidances, defenses, and contractions of awareness. Unconsciousness keeps a person stuck; mindfulness brings movement and growth.

When psychotherapy is founded on the principle of mindfulness, a number of implications and health values emerge for psychotherapy.

Here and Now

Grounding psychotherapy in mindfulness makes therapy present centered and shows how neurosis, wounding, and our defensive machinations take us out of the now. Indeed, psychological health can be seen as the degree to which a person is living in the present moment. All forms of psychological impairment reduce present centeredness and involve us in fantasies of the past and future.

Gestalt and existential therapies have spearheaded a present-focused approach to psychotherapy. In seeing the present moment as all that exists, the past is seen to exist here and now in the form of memory, recall, history, and nostalgia. The future is seen to exist here and now in the form of anticipation, hope, dread, despair, and fantasy. When we remember the past or anticipate the future, we do so *now*. Memory and anticipation are experienced now, and both past and future are present constructions of thought.

In psychotherapy, which deals extensively with how past wounding affects our current functioning, the past is seen to be present now in the form of unfinished emotional business, incomplete situations that continue to be unfinished in each present moment. These incomplete *gestalten* fester below the surface, clamoring for attention, drawing our energy away from the present moment. When psychotherapy addresses these unhealed wounds so they become healed in the present, the energy invested in them then becomes available for current life concerns. Slowly, over time, working through "old" business and the defenses that keep them out of awareness brings about greater living in the here and now. Another dimension of this sees psychological problems resulting from developmental fixations—fixations that occurred historically but are still continuing in the present. When therapy focuses on reactivating old developmental derailments, the client's growth process takes up where it had been and continues to be stuck. Attending to this remobilizes the client's natural movement forward, so growth resumes once again.

Coming into the now extends to the therapeutic relationship. With a temporal focus on the present, the transference is seen to be a present manifestation of past relationships, for the past is alive in how the client constructs and interprets the relationship with the therapist moment to moment. The person of the therapist also needs to be included in this understanding of the transference, for the actual behavior of the therapist significantly influences what is evoked in the transference. This is exactly the direction in which depth psychotherapy has moved over the last 20 years, and a present-centered orientation makes the actual here-and-now relationship with the client even more salient.

Focus on Actual Lived Experience

The experience of atman or Buddha-nature shows just how lost in thoughts, images, and fantasies most people are nearly all of the time. Ordinary experience consists of layers and layers of thoughts, memories, feelings, impulses, desires, fantasies, and other mental constructions that prevent us from living in actual, vivid contact with our senses and inner being. The practice of witness consciousness seeks to eliminate these filters, but its effects are quite limited for most people. Psychotherapy has discovered why this is so, namely, because a great deal of this virtual reality consists of compensations for painful feelings and early wounds that require a psychotherapeutic healing to truly resolve. Sustained mindfulness practice can reduce it for a period of time, but it is not possible for most people to live their lives in a meditation retreat. Psychotherapeutic working through, however, can have long-lasting effects and can clear out major areas of thought and fantasy preoccupation.

The meditative focus on actual, lived experience coincides nicely with existential therapy's agenda to uncover experience as it is, without preconceptions and an overlay of theories and therapeutic images. Coming out of European philosophy, especially existentialism and phenomenology, existential psychotherapy strongly distrusts theories and mere theorizing. As helpful as such approaches as psychoanalysis can be, theoretical structures can also become a kind of Procrustean bed in which the client is stretched or shrunk to fit the theory. By "bracketing off" preconceptions and metaphysical beliefs, phenomenologically informed therapy seeks to uncover experience just as it is. In encouraging a client to engage his or her experience fully, awareness is brought to a client's defenses and avoidances in working them through.

When we live in our heads in this virtual reality in which most people live, we are not in touch with actual reality. It is part of the shift away from the body into the mind as a defensive maneuver. This brings us to the next value.

Sensory and Organismic Involvement

Witness consciousness brings us into the body. Integrating mindfulness into psychotherapy means awakening the senses and eliciting a fuller engagement with our body, our breath, and our organismic aliveness. Gestalt therapy founder Fritz Perls used to exhort, "Lose your mind and come to your senses!" (Perls, 1969). When we leave the virtual reality of our mental constructions, we come into our body.

As consciousness "wakes up" through the process of attending to the immediacy of our experience in the moment, there is a greater perception of the felt sense emerging out of bodily experiencing. This shift into coming back into our body once again opens the vistas and richness of sensory experience. The glory of sight with its colors and textures, the beauty of hearing and tuning into our background auditory environment, the pleasure of sensing our body in movement or at rest—the body lives in the present, and in waking up we wake up to bodily experiencing.

The Being Dimension of Therapy

Health comes from Being, from the original wholeness that underlies the psyche. In this perspective, the person is whole *now*. Wholeness is not something to be achieved but is already here and immediately available if we can open to it. There is an infinite reservoir of untapped capacity and potential enfolded in Being, and in opening to this part of ourselves we discover we have the resources to deal with whatever situation with which we are faced. The Buddhist concept of "intrinsic health" corresponds to this notion, for just beneath our pain and uncertainty is the radical aliveness of the ground of consciousness.

The key is "being with" our experience. Rather than pushing or manipulating ourselves and trying to be somehow different than we are, this approach encourages us to simply accept and be with whatever feelings and issues with which we are struggling. In this act of being with, we are relating to ourselves in a different way, no longer pushing away or recoiling from ourselves. In being with ourselves and staying with our experience, our experience deepens and moves us naturally toward greater resolution.

There are different strategies for relating to ourselves by "being with" our experience. First is the gestalt method of *being* it—becoming the anger or fear or whatever problematic feeling wih which we are struggling. In no longer resisting it but identifying with it completely, the feeling begins to open up and reveal itself, taking us deeper within. Another approach is not to be it but to *lean into* it, to touch it but stay apart from it, listening and sensing the feeling, letting it speak. In this second way we maintain a slight separation from the feeling or impulse but gently tap on it to see what it is. A third poise of consciousness is to stand back from the feeling, to *detach and observe it* from a little distance, to disidentify from it and see it as different than oneself. In this third way, which can be especially helpful in trauma or with feelings that are difficult to tolerate, the distance allows the person to feel safe and not overwhelmed by the problematic feelings. Yet in observing and feeling them from a distance, the person opens to whatever the feelings bring, allowing them to move through and complete themselves.

Each of these stances involves a different relationship to emotion: fully identified with, close to, or more distant from. Each person has easier access to emotional experience by "being with" feelings in one or another of these ways. A mindfulness approach to therapy can utilize all of these to see what works best for a given client. Ideally, the client will move toward a flexible stance that can relate to feelings from anywhere along this continuum of identification as the situation demands.

Silence and Nonverbal Being

Mindfulness practice values nonverbal experiencing. The atman (or Buddha-nature) is a silent, ever-peaceful ground beyond all words and thought. The thinking mind, even when thinking about profound issues, is a more superficial level of consciousness than the ground of atman. Very often, interpersonal anxiety compels us to fill the air with words and chatter, preventing us from appreciating silence and a nonverbal level of being. Words and compulsive talking are ways of dealing with and sometimes moving through anxiety, but they also can perpetuate anxiety and keep us at a more surface level of experience. When we invite a deepening of awareness into nonverbal realms, we see how much our words act as barriers to experiencing. As experience deepens (in therapy or meditation), we come closer to this silent core of our being. There is a wisdom inherent in deeper being, which we can then experience as we enter into this deeper peace and silence. Entering into a deeper, nonverbal mode of being opens up a new appreciation for words and verbal communication. Verbalization is most effective when it flows out of Being rather than being compulsive chatter that blocks deeper experiencing.

Acceptance of Whatever Arises

Mindfulness practice means accepting whatever emerges, without defense or judgment. In mindfulness meditation, the instruction is to nonreactively accept whatever arises in consciousness, to observe it carefully, and to witness it passing away. This implies a good deal of nondefensiveness. The problem, of course, is that our unconscious defenses operate no matter what, even when we try to stop ourselves from judging or justifying or defending.

Depth psychotherapy is the first psychological method developed to decrease defensiveness. Mindfulness meditation practice, although it may penetrate defensive structures temporarily in some moments, does not actually work through defenses and allow them to drop away. Psychotherapy, on the other hand, engages defenses directly through confrontation and indirectly through eroding defenses over time in the accepting, empathic atmosphere of the therapeutic relationship. Mindfulness can support this process and can even carry it farther, encouraging therapist and client to let go of all preconceptions about what should arise in awareness. Acceptance then leads directly to taking responsibility for our experience, a key therapeutic value. Responsibility flows out of acceptance, in that once we accept a given feeling or experience, we can then claim it as our own and respond appropriately to it. Responsibility does not mean blame; it means ownership and claiming personal experience.

Presence

As we progressively let go of defenses, avoidances, and inauthentic modes of being, and as we complete unfinished business from the past so that more of our authentic self comes into, we come more fully into the present and experience greater presence. Presence comes as we wake up into the present. We feel more centered, more connected to the ground of our being, and more of us is available. We feel more "there," more responsive, more aware of our own depths. As our relationship to our self deepens, we can connect to others at a deeper level. The depth of our intimate relationships is limited only by how deeply we are connected to ourselves.

In awakening to the present and becoming more aware of the ego and its defenses, consciousness is able to go deeper within. New interior spaces open up, new vistas of inner being. We touch into a deeper authenticity, our essential nature or intrinsic self, our *svabhava* as it manifests in our frontal being. This is connected to our deeper inner being—inner mind, inner vital, inner (subtle) physical—which has a direct contact with the cosmic and universal forces. We then come to the *purusha* or witness consciousness. Usually it is the mental *purusha* or true mental being that is first contacted. This is the delegate of the atman on this plane, and it is a silent, pure observer detached from all contents. This witness consciousness can be accessed immediately, at any time, although, as one Tibetan Buddhist teacher has stated, almost no one can stay in this experience for more than a few seconds. Nevertheless, in tapping into this witness consciousness, a new dimension of awareness becomes available that deepens presence still farther. Going beyond this witness consciousness or true mental being, the psychic center is the inmost level, though this is virtually an unknown dimension of consciousness.

Western psychology generally stops at the level of the observing ego and the authentic self. Existential therapy moves in the direction of Being but stops short at a finite being, the limited person. Though this being is the border to a greater inner Being, very few approaches move beyond. Ali's diamond approach, Jungian psychology, and psychosynthesis go farther into the inner being and true being but still stop short of the psychic being. The inner space that opens up in these interior realms is often conflated with other realms, and there is much confusion about the sense of space, emptiness, and void that is encountered in these deeper levels. However, the deeper within consciousness one can travel, the greater the sense of Being and presence becomes.

In entering into the inner world, a new appreciation of aloneness emerges. For the surface consciousness, loneliness is a great problem.

The frontal self is fundamentally relational, and when the self is deprived of relationships for very long, it experiences a state of deficiency and lack, a longing for contact with others, and a sense of its own insufficiency. The feeling of loneliness is hard to bear and makes many people flee into escapes, drugs, and inauthentic living to cope with this hard, existential reality. However, when the inner life opens up, the experience of loneliness changes.

Being alone, rather than something to be avoided, becomes something valuable and nourishing. The initial feeling of inner deficiency and emptiness that meets the surface consciousness opens into a vastness when we stay with it rather than avoid it. Lonely insufficiency and lack can give way to a sense of fullness and inward richness as the inner being is accessed. Though contact with others remains essential to nourish the frontal self, there can be a greater independence and inner support as consciousness opens within. This greater freedom can then devolve into a rationale for avoiding relationships, and so it can become another form of spiritual bypassing when schizoid tendencies and avoidant attachment patterns are not therapeutically worked through. But with a psychologically attuned person, deepening presence can dramatically transform the experience of loneliness.

Vulnerability and Power

The Western image of power is a kind of John Wayne, macho "toughness." This image is held out by contemporary culture as a symbol of strength, while vulnerability is often equated to being weak or fragile. But in the context of psychotherapy, vulnerability means openness to experience. There is great power in being open to our own deeper being, for this is our ground and true support. In fact, a depth exploration of a typical "macho" toughness reveals that this façade hides an interior fragility and anxiety. The "tough" exterior is often a rigid set of contractions, a closed, shut-down, constricted shield against life's blows that betrays a deeper sense of fear and powerlessness.

The capacity to be open, vulnerable, exposed to others, and accepting of tender, soft, or even dark and shameful feelings takes great courage. To be able to rest in our own emotional experience, to be grounded in our fundamental openness to the world without barriers or defenses, is a stance of immense power, for we are then rooted in our depths, unshaken by passing storms on the surface. As Krishnamurti (1958) put it, "To be vulnerable is to live, to withdraw is to die." We are powerful when we can be vulnerable and open—whether we are open to tears or anger or love, for we then stand firmly in the power of our emotional truth. This vulnerability is a power that can triumph over all outer failures and defeats, for then we can flexibly cope with life and move on.

Clarity

Clear seeing dissolves our unconscious conditioning and reactivity. This clarity or movement of insight is a function of our deeper nature, atman, or Buddha-mind. Witness consciousness brings us into a larger, more expanded consciousness that has an inward spaciousness. As the outer, surface mind settles down into interior silence, it opens to a creative, fertile void that clearly sees whatever arises, like a mirror that reflects with pristine clarity what is put before it.

APPLICATIONS OF MINDFULNESS IN PSYCHOTHERAPY

There are general and specific applications of mindfulness practice to psychotherapy. Humanistic and existential psychotherapies were the first to be significantly influenced by Eastern mindfulness practices. There is a great similarity of language between Buddhism and gestalt therapy, for example, and between existentialism and Taoism. Hakomi (Kurtz, 1990) shows how mindfulness can be used in somatic work. In the past decades, mindfulness practice, especially in the form of Buddhism, has entered into the psychoanalytic literature (see, e.g., Epstein, 1996; Rubin, 1996; Engler, 1986). The therapeutic and health values discussed earlier have begun to find their way into psychoanalytic thinking and have become an important countervailing influence against the focus on pathology and past-centered orientation that has typified much of traditional analytic work.

Specific applications of mindfulness principles have emerged in two well-known approaches. Linehan's (1993) dialectical behavior therapy uses mindfulness as a cornerstone in working with borderline personality disorders and now has considerable research validation behind it that substantiates it as an effective methodology. Kabat-Zinn (1990) has brought mindfulness practice into the area of stress reduction and pain management with equally impressive results. These two examples show how mindfulness methods can be integrated into specific treatment approaches in psychotherapy.

A number of therapeutic strategies for becoming more mindful and present-centered are used by different schools. These include the following:

- completing old, unfinished business
- unfolding present potentials of the self, favored by existential approaches
- bringing old, buried, undeveloped aspects of the self on-line by completing interrupted developmental processes and filling in deficits in self-structure, favored by psychodynamic approaches
- behavioral prescriptions to act now to replace avoidance with exposure to what is feared and expanding behavioral possibilities
- coming into the body, both sensorily and emotionally, through the bodily felt sense, an approach used by somatic therapies
- coming into the here and now in the transference, an approach pioneered by existential therapy and now gaining wide acceptance in analytic circles
- reducing fantasy by enhancing sensory experience, or else using fantasy as a gateway to working with emotional issues
- confronting defenses or having them erode through empathic acceptance, as defenses drop away, more present-centeredness results
- stopping addictive distractions and replacing them with genuine, real satisfactions, that is, developing a more cohesive self whose needs are more fully met rather than being lost in daydreams or fantasies
- letting go of inauthentic ways of being by seeing how they are avoidances of difficult issues and affects, choosing and creating new, authentic ways of being that enhance aliveness and mindful living

Although these therapeutic strategies increase mindfulness, mindfulness is both the goal and the method. Bringing increased mindfulness to bear on these issues increases the power of the therapeutic process.

Two important limitations of mindfulness practice need to be acknowledged. The first is that mindfulness is a kind of "uncovering" technique that works in the direction of unmasking or exposing defenses. For most psychotherapy clients who are at a neurotic level of functioning, this is precisely what is needed. However, with more severe psychological disturbances, especially with clients who may be psychotic, structure-building techniques are generally regarded as more appropriate, since uncovering techniques can be disorganizing and fragmenting. However, this is not a hard-and-fast rule. For a long time it was believed that mindfulness practices were contraindicated for borderline personality disorders (see Engler, 1986) for the same reason that they could be disorganizing. However, Linehan's (1993) work demonstrates that mindfulness can be utilized quite effectively with this population, illustrating that it is better not to come to a premature conclusion about this.

The second caution about mindfulness practice involves its focus on mind rather than feeling. In the meditation world, practitioners of mindfulness practice can easily fall into the trap of becoming clear but cool—aware of thoughts and sensations but subtly and unconsciously using mindfulness as a kind of super-ego judging and way to detach from difficult affects and unpleasant emotions. Although this goes against the fundamental guidelines for mindfulness meditation, in actual practice this is difficult to avoid unless there is considerable psychological work to undo the defensive avoidances of feeling. In psychotherapeutic practice, this same tendency can arise. There can be the appearance of mindfulness of inner states, while in reality problematic emotions are only glancingly felt and dispensed with rather than gone into and fully experienced.

Despite these limitations, mindfulness is a powerful practice for exploring consciousness. It is in one sense the fundamental "method" of all depth psychotherapy, "making the unconscious conscious" as Freud first put it, but it illumines areas of consciousness that go far beyond Western psychological maps and opens up the spiritual foundation of consciousness. When brought into a psychotherapeutic context, it makes psychotherapy a form of meditation, both for the client and the therapist.

DOING PSYCHOTHERAPY AS
MINDFULNESS PRACTICE

The process of being a psychotherapist involves inner psychological work first and foremost, for only by engaging our own healing at a deep level can we help others deeply engage their own healing. This principle also holds true for integrating mindfulness practice into psychotherapy. It begins with the therapist's practice of mindfulness.

When the therapist is established in an ongoing, serious practice of mindfulness, then the process of doing psychotherapy becomes an extension of this. In paying attention to the mind's activity—the endless chatter, associations, images, and sensations—a gradual calming occurs over time. Sustained attention and practice result in an inward deepening as consciousness wakes up into its own interior spaces. In becoming more centered in our own depths, we relate to doing psychotherapy differently. There is a kind of depth perception that comes where it is possible to see more deeply into the client, to empathically grasp the client's experience more fully. Mindfully observing our own consciousness extends outward, so the therapist is better able to attend to the client's experience. In coming into direct relationship with ourselves, we come into better contact with the client.

Witness consciousness results in a greater sense of being centered, calm, and less reactive. No one can expect to be a perfect Buddha, silent and without emotional responses, but with practice, greater equanimity, steadiness, and clear seeing are within reach. Practicing psychotherapy then becomes the practice of mindfulness. We can meet the client more completely, because we are more awake and more present inwardly.

Greater presence on the part of the therapist in turn facilitates the therapeutic process. The therapist's mindfulness creates an atmosphere that profoundly influences the process of psychotherapy. While the receptivity of the client is important, and the mutual influence of the client's consciousness on the therapist must be included, the greater the therapist's presence, the more effective the therapy will tend to be.

Chapter 7

Psychotherapy As Opening the Heart
Bhakti Yoga

Your vision will become clear only when you can look into your own heart.
Who looks outside, dreams; who looks inside, awakes.

—Carl Jung

The third traditional point of entry to the inner world is through the heart. Psychotherapy and spirituality can be seen to have the same goal: *opening the heart*. Both seek to expand the heart's capacity for feeling and love, but they proceed in very different ways. Spiritual traditions work to open the heart *directly*—through devotion, love, bhakti, positive emotions, and disidentifying with negative emotions. Psychotherapy, on the other hand, works to open the heart by *seeing how it is closed*—by exploring the defenses against feelings and by reowning painful, negative emotions, the avoidance of which so limits the heart's emotional range.

The heart closes in several specific ways that have now been studied in great detail. Psychotherapy and spiritual practice work to open the heart once again. But before examining how a synthesis of these two approaches can open the heart fully and integrally, let us first examine how psychology and spirituality work on their own.

PSYCHOTHERAPY AS OPENING THE HEART

The history of psychology can be read as a dawning recognition of the heart as the key to psychological life. Modern psychology began with

125

Freud showing just how much the mind is at the mercy of powerful, unconscious feelings and instincts, a puppet whose strings are continually pulled by emotional forces. As psychoanalysis evolved and the self came into better focus, it has become even clearer how essential emotions are for psychological functioning. Affects and affect regulation are now seen as central functions of the self.

The last few decades have seen important advances in research, especially in the fields of affect theory, emotion research, attachment theory, and neuroscience. These scientific developments confirm what the depth psychology schools have maintained for some time, namely, that *feelings are essential guides in life.*

Of the vast amount of information coming into the brain, there needs to be a way to order it, to prioritize what is important and what is not. Emotion is the central way of organizing our brain and consciousness. If this organization is disorganized and incoherent, then our life is in disorder, with great suffering and pain. But if it is coherent, clear, and in good order, then life is joyous and fulfilling. *Organizing, modulating, and regulating emotion is the key.*

When a therapist asks a client in psychotherapy, "What does this mean to you?" the therapist is asking, in effect, "What are your feelings about this?" *Feelings are inseparable from meaning.* Meaning also contains a cognitive component, but it is the affective dimension that makes an experience meaningful. Recent research in neuroscience has discovered that the way a person establishes meaning is closely linked to social interactions. This is understandable, because *the heart comes online through relationships.* Thus, meaning and interpersonal experience are connected, because they are mediated by the same neural circuits responsible for emotion (Siegel, 1999; Schore, 1999, 2003.) Feelings, meaning, and interpersonal experience are intimately linked. This is why deep psychological change, in the self and in the neurological organization of the brain, requires an intense interpersonal experience such as that which occurs in the therapeutic relationship.

Emotions organize our experience in four basic ways:

1. as *information*
2. as a way of *evaluating* situations
3. as a form of *communication*
4. as a *direction for our behavior*

Feelings give us information about people and the world that we get in no other way. At the simplest level, emotions tell us what is good or bad, nourishing or toxic, and they make this evaluation rapidly, without a long, logical process of reasoning. Feelings also are a means of communicating with others and of expressing ourselves, a way we see others and are seen by them. Additionally, feelings motivate us to take the next step forward in our lives, giving us a guiding direction for how to act to best meet our needs.

Affect theory and emotion research study the universals of emotional life. Through rigorous research with infants and adults across cultures, psychologists have discovered that certain basic affects appear to be hardwired into the human brain. Infants from around the world universally express these basic affects shortly after birth. Every culture throughout the world displays these basic emotions through identical facial expressions and voice quality, although cultures vary in their degree of expressiveness.

The field of emotion research identifies eight basic emotions: joy, interest and excitement, caring and love, fear, shame, anger, disgust, and sadness and despair. These then combine, refine, and further differentiate into an endless variety of feeling states. As we develop emotionally, we experience increasing richness, subtlety, and differentiation in our emotional life, which will continue to evolve throughout our entire life.

The first three of the basic eight emotions often are called "positive" emotions and the last five "negative." Of course, since all emotions help us creatively adapt, they are all positive in that sense. "Positive" or "negative" feelings generally refer to how people experience them, as pleasant or unpleasant. It is theorized that there has been an evolutionary advantage in having a greater differentiation of negative feelings, allowing a greater chance for survival. For example, it is adaptive to feel fear as a lion approaches and to run away to safety, or to feel anger and to fight off an aggressor. These feelings increase a person's chances for survival.

Just because there are more negative feelings than positive ones does not mean we should feel negative more often; just the opposite is true. When we are living in alignment with our authentic nature, we generally feel a preponderance of joy, warmth, and positive feelings of interest and engagement in our life. If we do not and instead feel primarily negative feelings, this is a signal that something is wrong. We are not paying attention to something in our life. Our feelings are telling us that something needs to change

Feelings allow us to navigate the complex interpersonal world in which we all live. They help us evaluate situations. By magnifying what is positive or negative in our experience, feelings are *experience amplifiers*. For example, in eating rotting food, the unpleasant smell and taste are amplified by the feeling of disgust, which causes us to expel it quickly, something that also had great survival value for our ancestors. This led affect researcher Sylvan Tomkins (1963) to note that feelings make good things better and bad things worse.

Without feelings, we have no basis for knowing what is important or what is irrelevant, who we can trust or mistrust, or who we can love or avoid. Are we moving in the right direction in life? Are we with the right people who nourish and support us, or are we choosing unhealthy relationships that poison and deplete us? Only our heart can tell us.

Neuroscience researchers have discovered that people who have a brain injury that eliminates their capacity to sense their feelings while leaving their mental abilities unimpaired suffer a great disability in living. Without our feelings to evaluate which options are best, life is an overwhelming array of choices. Logic alone is insufficient. When all options are possible, the mind spins off into hundreds of possibilities, but it has nothing to anchor it. Without feelings, we are lost.

Feelings allow us to communicate emotionally with others. Our heart allows us to read other people emotionally and, in turn, to be read by them. Our emotional awareness tunes us into what others are feeling, adjusts our feeling state appropriately, and signals back to others what we are feeling. For example, a mother gently nursing her baby creates an unmistakable joy that the baby expresses through smiling blissfully, relaxing, and gurgling with pleasure. This makes the mother feel good and loving, and it reinforces her taking care of her baby, ensuring that the baby gets the nurturing it needs.

Neuroscience has discovered that a key part of the brain that processes emotion is the "mammalian brain" or limbic system that we share with other mammals, though not with reptiles and lower life-forms. The warm, emotional bond between a dog and its owner, for example, transcends species. In contrast, any bond between a snake and its owner will be strictly one-way.

Ideally our feelings guide us toward love, growth, and self-fulfillment. But as depth psychology has long known and recent infant research in attachment theory has confirmed, our early childhood wounding leads us far astray. Attachment theory studies mother-infant bonding and how these early attachment patterns persist over a lifetime. Attachment research shows how the heart's guidance develops *through relationship*. It is our attachment to our earliest caregivers that brings forth our emotional intelligence.

Since feeling life begins with the first relationships with the mother and father, an empathic, loving atmosphere is necessary to affirm the child's feelings so he or she can own them. Ideally the infant attaches to a mother and father who are loving, responsive, and empathically attuned. This secure base allows the growing child to relate the heart's feelings to a context of genuine love and attuned caring, setting up a lifelong pattern of being able to choose people who are truly nourishing. Unfortunately, this never happens perfectly and usually goes far astray. The pervasive wounding that affects every person on the planet distorts this process to some degree.

Feelings that are met with anxiety or shame by the parents are soon driven underground. All feelings that are threatening to the parents (due to their childhood wounding) are pushed into the unconscious. The first priority of any child is maintaining the attachment to the mother and father. This relationship must be protected at all costs. Any feelings that threaten this relationship are shut down, limiting the child's access to feelings. We erect unconscious defenses against our own feelings so that we no longer even know what our feelings are. Little by little, the heart closes. Its guiding light dims.

Research into attachment theory clearly documents how early childhood wounding constricts our attention and keeps us stuck in rigid patterns. We look for love along the familiar grooves that we originally experienced in our family, setting us up to reenact the same repetitive patterns from childhood that frustrated and hurt us as children. We become attracted to lovers and friends who are emotionally unavailable in the same way our parents and family were. With many repetitions and reinforcements, the neural pathways grow stronger as the brain develops. Neuroscience has established how early conditioning becomes more entrenched in the brain's neurological structure. We keep trying to master this old, frustrating situation, but unfortunately these attempts usually keep us repeating it with only minor variations. As the heart closes, our ability to relate shrinks, and we move in smaller and smaller circles. This does not self-correct on its own but requires some kind of intervention to change, which research shows can be accomplished in psychotherapy. This is an example from my clinical practice:

> In his early 30's, Richard entered therapy for depression. He didn't know why he was depressed or even what many of his feelings were. He only knew he felt bad and was estranged from his friends and work. His depression began after he ended his third unsuccessful relationship with a woman he found "smothering." At the start of their relationship, Richard had been attracted by her independent spirit. Yet soon after they got together, he reported, this began to change. She became more needy and clingy. Richard found himself letting go of other friendships so they could spend more and more time together.
>
> This was a familiar pattern in Richard's relationships. Even though he wanted to keep seeing his friends, he found himself irresistibly drawn into this relationship. At the beginning it was intensely passionate, but soon their sexual excitement began to wane. It seemed to Richard that the more he gave, the more she needed, until he spiraled down and down, feeling hopeless about either making her happy or feeling fulfilled himself in their relationship.
>
> The first period of therapy centered around Richard learning to better identify his different feelings and to more fully sense his bodily awareness of them. As his emotional world came into better focus, Richard was able to recognize the familiarity of his feelings and how they resonated with earlier feelings from long ago in his family. Richard's mother had been depressed and had looked to Richard to make her feel better. But no matter how hard Richard had tried to save his mother, it was more than he could manage. Richard was left feeling like a failure in letting his mother down but felt he had no other choice but to try still harder in this hopeless task.
>
> A turning point came as Richard connected deeply with the depleted, despairing little boy inside who had given up on

ever getting his needs met by his mother and who felt like something was wrong with him because he was unable to rescue his mother from her depression. Early depression around this revealed a complex of anger, hurt, shame, and grief that had been long banished because they jeopardized his relationship with his mother. As these early feelings were worked through, new parts of Richard began to emerge. His lifelong coping strategy of taking care of his partner gave way to a greater vitality and enthusiasm in his life, and he found himself attracted to new kinds of women, women who also could meet *his* needs in the dance of relationship.

As psychotherapy proceeds, defenses gradually melt away. In the safety of the therapeutic relationship, the heart progressively reemerges as feelings guide the working-through process.

Because of our wounding and our defenses against this wounding, the "normalcy" of living in our heads has become pervasive. Psychology shines a light on the immense unconsciousness of such "normal" living. The vast majority of people do not realize just how diminished their feeling sense is, or to what extent they are moved in all of their actions by their heart's impulse. The crippled, shriveled heart that results from even a "normal" childhood severely impairs the wisdom of our heart's guidance. If we do not know our own heart, then how can we recognize true love?

Psychotherapy changes this *by undoing blocks*. It brings about self-acceptance by working through shame. We come to feel healthy self-love by working through our self-hate. We discover how to have loving relationships in the present by working through frustrating, rejecting relationships from the past. Psychotherapy has discovered that we cannot go higher than we can go low, so going into our pain, we increase our capacity for pleasure. The flow of feeling increases as we stop constricting it. The heart opens by exploring how it is shut down.

At a basic existential level, all human beings feel a great deal of fear and loneliness simply in being alive. Finding love and companionship is essential to all of us at this level. Further, unless we find intrinsically interesting work, we feel alienated and either bored or stressed, or both. It is no wonder that we then try to distract ourselves by escaping from what seems to be the emptiness and futility of existence. But in removing the defenses and blocks around the heart, escapes become unnecessary. Closing the heart imprisons the authentic self; opening the heart liberates it. *There is no other way of self-finding than by way of the heart.*

THE OPENING FROM PSYCHOTHERAPY

As the heart opens, the false self dissipates and the authentic self comes forth. Our authentic self has a wide range of emotional capacities essential for a good life, one that is richly textured with rewarding personal relationships, creative work, and deep meaning. The authentic self develops to some degree the following 20 abilities, which comprise the essence of emotional intelligence:

1. The authentic self has access to the full range of basic feelings—joy, interest, affection, fear, shame, anger, disgust, and sadness.

2. The authentic self can feel the full range of intensities of feelings rather than a very limited range (for example, rather than only feeling mild irritation and then later on exploding, we are able to feel all of the different intensities of anger, from mild irritation to annoyance to moderate anger, up through rage and volcanic, white-hot fury).

3. Emotional awareness includes how the mind symbolizes emotional experience. We learn to identify our feelings and have a mental understanding or cognitive schema of different feelings.

4. We become better at verbally and nonverbally expressing our feelings skillfully in the variety of our relationships, such as lover, family, friend, coworker, and so on.

5. We can empathically tune into others' feeling states and recognize and respond to their feelings.

6. We are able to *express* or *contain* feelings as appropriate, without resorting either to acting them out or repressing them.

7. We develop the capacity to self-soothe and calm ourselves, to modulate feelings of anxiety or distress internally without resorting to external means such as alcohol, drugs, or food. We can regulate our affects without being overwhelmed or overstimulated by them.

8. Everyone struggles with a split between tender and sexual feelings. Psychotherapy works to unite tender and sexual feelings toward the same person. Another split is good and bad, seeing another person as all good one moment and all bad later on. Therapy works to end this splitting into good and bad and achieving object constancy, the perception of one whole person.

9. We can "go with" our feelings—to flow with emotional experience and allow the feeling process to unfold (for example, feeling the grief fully after a loss, intensely at first, then decreasing in intensity over time, and eventually being finished with it).

10. We can go deeper into our feelings to see what they connect to in the past. This involves an awareness of incomplete gestalts as we "peel the onion" of emotional experience. We get a better handle on our reactivity or emotional buttons so that we can work with past unfinished situations when they are activated by present events.

11. We have an observing ego and are able to observe our feelings nonreactively, a witness consciousness that prevents us from being carried away and lost in feelings. This does not mean becoming dissociated or overly detached under the guise of witnessing.

12. We get a handle on our own defensiveness and are able to recognize it and work with it, dealing with the underlying threats to our self-esteem and self-cohesion.

13. We are guided by our feelings rather than by introjected shoulds or internalized authority (for example, forgiveness emerging naturally after having worked through our anger rather than forcing forgiveness out of a should or an ideal).

14. We become more conscious of how feelings live in the body, including awareness of the felt sense, the breath, and the energetic experience of emotion. We can breathe freely to support emotional experience, letting the strength of feelings move the breath (for example, breathing deeply during high arousal states, such as sexual activity or intense anger or crying).

15. We are able to develop, maintain, and deepen a whole range of relationships to meet our emotional needs. These include

relationships with people who fundamentally love and affirm us; people we look up to, admire, and respect (including teachers and mentors who can provide guidance); colleagues and coworkers we feel competent around; a lover or sexual partner with whom we feel a special bond of intimacy and love; and friends with whom we feel completely comfortable and around whom we can be ourselves.

16. We can sense how feelings are symbolized in the mind through fantasy, images, symbols, and words.

17. We become more resilient and better able to bounce back after life's inevitable emotional setbacks and shocks. We can form and make use of a support system for emotional sustenance and nurturing.

18. Our emotional life develops toward greater complexity, differentiation, subtlety, and richness. We cultivate the heart and refine the feeling capacity so it unfolds from primitive, archaic levels toward greater maturity and depth.

19. We can move between spontaneity and controlled deliberateness as appropriate. Neurosis involves overcontrol and lack of spontaneity. Other personality organizations such as borderline conditions involve lack of control. Life demands both capacities, and freedom consists in being able to shift between "letting go" and "being deliberate" as the situation demands.

20. Increasing freedom from early family patterns in our relationships. We develop new ways of relating to others that reflect our increasing sense of realness, authenticity, and aliveness.

As the authentic self emerges more fully, it has access to these emotional abilities of the heart. Our heart is continuously giving us feedback about the people around us, our interactions, our present environment, our past, and our future directions. Our heart's guidance is profound and essential for full living.

Psychology has discovered that through the process of feeling we can disentangle ourselves from the snares of inauthentic living. By following our heart's true impulse, we find our way toward authenticity. Our authentic self seeks to fulfill itself on every level—physical, lower emotional, central emotional, higher emotional, and mental. It needs the world to bring forth its full powers—an awakened body sense that reveals the embodied richness of living, love and intimate connection and nourishing relationships of all kinds, freedom of the imagination and creativity, and mental stimulation and meaningful work to express the self's true talents. It is only the heart's radical aliveness that reveals the richness and intensity that come when these things are part of our life.

Using our heart's guidance to find what we need for "the good life" represents a major step forward in evolution. But as revolutionary as greater authenticity is for human welfare, the human spirit requires more. As discussed earlier, psychology leads to our outer authentic nature (*svabhava*) but not our inner authentic nature. An authentic life is a major development, but it is not enough. Psychology alone does not give us a vision of a higher life. In our heart of hearts, our deepest soul longs for more.

SPIRITUALITY AS OPENING THE HEART

Spirituality has a very different view of opening the heart, and it proceeds in quite a different way. Spirituality brings forth our true soul or psychic center. In the traditional religious view, it is our psychological material that covers up the soul's deeper light. Spirituality tries to separate out this emotional dross from the pure gold that shines out from the soul. Spirituality works to directly open the inner doors of the heart through love, aspiration, and positive feelings while detaching from their opposites. The very feelings that psychology sees as grist for the mill, spirituality regards as impediments to an open heart. Spirituality uses the higher, more refined emotions of love, devotion, aspiration, bhakti, surrender, and adoration to purify and refine the consciousness so the soul's light can shine forth.

Rather than simply bringing about new emotional capacities as psychology does, spirituality brings forth a *new dimension of consciousness.* Just as the heart discloses another realm of consciousness than body consciousness can provide, and just as mind opens to a level of consciousness beyond the heart, so the soul or psychic center unveils another dimension of consciousness. This new consciousness permeates and infuses our current physical, emotional, and mental levels of being and opens up something infinitely more and immeasurably precious. It is an inner light that entirely changes our experience of living.

When the lotus of the heart breaks open, we feel a divine joy, love and peace expanding in us like a flower of light which irradiates the whole being. (Aurobindo, 1973b, p. 570)

When the psychic center or soul awakens, we open to a self-existent joy, a concrete, palpable sense of bliss that is ever present, ever fresh, like an eternal spring eternally bubbling forth with an utter peace and happiness. No matter what our external circumstances, this inner fount of joy is ever available within.

This spring of joy also is a source of the sweetest love, a love that simply *is*. This love is not dependent on any outer situations or stimulation but is intrinsic to the soul's nature. It is a continual unfolding of the most sublime affection that gives an extraordinary perfume to life and extends out into the world.

Discernment is a further characteristic of the psychic center. Because it comes from the Divine Truth, it has an inherent truth sense and an unerring guidance. It provides a discrimination (*viveka*) and a sense of the world beyond the mind's reasonings. Because the outer is an expression of the inner, that is, because the self is an expression of the evolving soul, the soul is the self's true real guide. It the evolutionary element within, and only the psychic center can show us the way toward our future evolution.

The heart becomes a radiant center of inner guidance and joyous love, and much of the world's spiritual literature is an ecstatic poem to this happy state. As the psychic center awakens, such a person becomes "a friend to all creatures," says Krishna in the *Gita*. The sweetness of divine love surpasses even the highest bliss of earthly love, of which it is a reduced, stepped-down version. Relationships become a rapturous, loving encounter with the Divine's infinite forms as the world transforms into the soul's sacred playground.

This veiled psychic entity is the flame of the Godhead always alight within us, inextinguishable even by that dense unconsciousness of any spiritual self within which obscures our outer nature. It is a flame born out of the Divine and, luminous inhabitant of the Ignorance, grows in it till it is able to turn it towards the Knowledge. It is the concealed Witness and Control, the hidden Guide, the inner light or inner voice of the mystic. It is that which endures and is imperishable in us from birth to birth, untouched by death, decay or corruption, an indestructible spark of the Divine. . . . This psychic entity points always towards Truth and Right and Beauty, towards Love and Harmony and all this is a divine possibility within us, and persists till these things become the major need of our nature. (Aurobindo, 1970, p. 225)

Generally, all of these effects do not appear fully and immediately. More often it is a gradual coming forth of these qualities, like the dawning of the sun. Three steps forward often are followed by two steps back, as we assimilate these inner changes, but the movement is progressively forward. Though we may be pulled outward and away from it at times during the day, the psychic center is ever inwardly awake.

We are unconscious of our deeper soul, however, because in growing up and developing as a separate ego, we are drawn outward by the senses and desire. In identifying with these surface activities, the self becomes alienated from the soul and its intimacy with the Divine. However, through spiritual practice this separation can be healed. The heart is the key.

Opening the heart is a developmental process.[1] Spiritual development begins with less pure devotion, love, and aspiration and grows into more pure and intense forms of these feelings. Both Eastern psychology and Western religion have developed essentially similar spiritual practices, although the outward form varies between cultures. The first stage of practice involves moral and ethical behavior, religious instruction, and the fellowship of seekers. These practices direct the person's attention toward what is important (spirit) and away from life's many distractions. This preliminary stage also calms the mind. It eliminates the grossest forms of disturbance and lays a foundation for more sustained devotion. The next stage of practice involves inner practices, such as meditation, prayer, surrender, and devotional rituals. This stage begins to awaken the inner consciousness that is normally veiled by ordinary life. It deepens devotion and increases the soul's thirst for God. In the third stage, outer practices drop away and are replaced by greater inwardness, devotion, and surrender. As the aspirant's practice continues, further concentration clears away remaining distractions, so heart and mind become progressively one-pointed. As devotion focuses the aspirant lovingly upon the Divine, the Divine draws the soul closer in an increasing intimacy toward ultimate union.

In India the path of the heart is known as bhakti yoga. Christianity's gospel of love is a form of bhakti yoga, and this devotional stream is prominent in Islam and Judaism as well. Christ is often pictured pointing to his radiant soul in the "sacred heart." St. Teresa of Avila describes God as "enthroned on our heart," an almost identical image to the *Bhagavad Gita*'s image of the "Lord abiding in the heart of all beings." Most of India is devotional, and the numerous schools of bhakti yoga envisage the Divine in myriad forms—male and female, such as Vishnu, Krishna, and Shiva, and many forms of the Divine Mother. The path of the heart is the most prevalent spiritual path throughout the world, for all theistic religions have a strong bhakti element.

Bhakti yoga views the Divine not only as an infinite impersonal consciousness but as a supremely personal Being. In nondual theistic traditions, love is the fundamental relationship of the Divine with all creation. Individual souls are a portion of this divine Being and partake of this divine reality through the relationship of love. It is not a merger and dissolution of the ego, as in the traditions of the Impersonal Divine, but a state of difference, even in unity. "I want to taste the sugar," said Ramakrishna, "I don't want to become the sugar."

Love of the Divine Presence beyond all form is one approach, but most traditions focus upon specific forms or images of the Divine. Vedanta describes six main forms of relationships that the seeker may enjoy with the Divine.

1. *The Divine Child:* Viewing the Divine as an infant or as a child, such as baby Jesus or baby Krishna, or Krishna as a young boy, elicits tender, caring feelings in the aspirant that increase and deepen through devotional practice.
2. *The Divine Father:* This is how Jesus looked upon God, as does much of Western religion.
3. *The Divine Mother:* This relation often feels more close and intimate than the relation of father. Ramakrishna is perhaps India's most well-known child of the Mother.
4. *The Divine Friend:* This is the form that Krishna takes in many Indian stories and poems. The devotee is the friend or

playmate of Krishna in his *lila* (play), which brings out the sweetness, playfulness, and equality of relation even in its inequality.

5. *The Divine Master:* Here the devotee is a servant of the Divine, surrendered to God's will and acting as an instrument of God's action in the world. Islam and Judaism feature this element strongly. In this path, action (karma yoga) becomes a way to express devotion. In India, Hanuman serves as the ideal servant of Ram (God) in the ancient story or the Ramayana.

6. *The Divine Lover or Beloved:* The highest relation in India also is the most intimate and passionate relationship possible—that of lover and beloved. This also figures in the Christian tradition through such saints as St. John of the Cross and St. Teresa of Avila. Here the human passion for the divine reaches its culmination, as lover and Beloved fuse in a blissful union of love.

The path of the heart uses the rhythm of separation and return, seeking and finding, losing and finding again to ignite and increase the heart's fire. At first the presence of the Beloved is intermittent. The infinite peace and fulfillment of the divine Presence contrast sharply to the pangs of separation and the sense of feeling bereft and empty when the Beloved departs. But this serves only to increase the fires of longing and the joy of being reunited. Deeper and deeper layers of impurity and desire for outward things are burned up in the purifying fire of love. The density and outwardness of ordinary life pale as the soul's inner relation with the Divine grows in fineness, light, peace, and devotion. This is another case from my practice:

Ellen entered therapy after four years of what she called "the dark night of the soul." She confessed that although her spiritual director assured her that she only needed more faith and prayer to get through her "dark night," one of her few friends had urged her to seek out another perspective on her painful life. It soon became clear that whatever spiritual process she might have been undergoing, she also was depressed. She was not in an intimate relationship, and her strong religious beliefs kept her life confined to a limited circle of activities, mostly church related.

Ellen tried earnestly "to do God's will" in the world. Though she had toyed with the idea of becoming a nun in her 20s, instead she became loosely affiliated with a church-related group. Now in her 40s, her work and relationships were centered around this spiritual community. Her images of God were rather harsh, a severe, judgmental Being whose will she was continually falling short of. Pleasures of the flesh were discouraged, for they led one astray from the path of prayer and purification.

As Ellen's story came out in therapy, it became clear why she was depressed. She had almost no sources of genuine emotional gratification in her life. She felt bored with her work in her spiritual community. Her friendships were confined to a few other women whose lives were as strict and tightly regulated as hers. She forever felt like a failure in her spiritual progress, though she kept hoping for someone to recognize her attainments. Her depression was a very healthy response from her deeper self, a cry from her unconscious to stop ignoring so many of her needs.

Ellen's family, not surprisingly, also was very religious and rigid. Her father was an angry, critical man who was continually berating Ellen's mother and Ellen herself for their shortcomings. Ellen's mother was a submissive woman who had been physically abused by her father as a child, and whose approval Ellen always sought but never received.

Over the course of a few years, Ellen worked through much of the early wounding in her family of origin. As she did so, her images of God changed as well, from a harsh, condemning figure that reflected her punishing father into God as a loving and an accepting Being whom to she could turn for strength and comfort. As her rigidity melted, she made more friends, began to explore the wider world beyond her community, and eventually became involved in an intimate relationship with another woman from a different religious community. Her spirituality, she felt, began to deepen once again, and she began to experience some breakthroughs in her practice.

A purely spiritual approach to opening the heart opens us up to spiritual realms undreamt of by psychology, but historically the cost has been to turn our back on the world. Traditional spirituality seeks heaven by abandoning the earth.

THE ESSENTIAL CONFLICT

Psychology and spirituality seem to be fundamentally different, even to run in opposite directions. What are we to make of these two very different approaches to opening the heart? Are we to feel and express our anger, or do we let it go and focus on forgiveness? Is sexual attraction good or bad? Should we explore our feelings of shame and self-hate or disidentify with them and focus on self-love? Do we uncover the roots of our anxiety or try to concentrate on bringing peace and calm into our self? Does the good life consist of cultivating positive feelings such as forgiveness and love, or is this a repressive strategy that leads to psychological disaster?

Why do psychology and spirituality look so very different? And why do they produce two very different heart openings? How can we reconcile these divergent, contradictory strategies?

The answer is that *psychology and spirituality open different hearts.* Or, perhaps more accurately, each opens different levels of the heart. These two diverse approaches reflect the dual nature of the heart.

> This ambiguity, these opposing appearances of depth and blindness are created by the double character of the human emotive being. For there is in front in man a heart of vital emotion similar to the animal's, if more variously developed. . . . This mixture of the emotive heart and the sensational hungering vital creates in man a false soul of desire. . . . But the true soul of man is not there; it is in the true invisible heart hidden in some luminous cave of the nature: there under some infiltration of the divine Light is our soul. . . . It is as this psychic being in him grows and the movements of the heart reflect its divinations and impulses that man becomes more and more aware of his soul, ceases to be a superior animal and, awakening to glimpses of the godhead within him, admits more and more its intimations of a deeper life. (Aurobindo, 1973b, p. 150)

The heart is a double center. In front is the heart that psychology studies, with all of its unconscious defenses and depths. Behind and deep within lies what the spiritual traditions speak of, our soul or psychic center. The failure to distinguish between these two dimensions of being is the cause of much confusion and seeming paradox. Psychology opens the frontal, outer levels of the heart but is utterly lost when it attempts to go farther. Spirituality opens the inner heart but creates chaos in applying its strategies to ordinary life and relationships.

The biggest problem with psychology is its limited vision of the human being—it embraces earth and ignores heaven. But without a larger, spiritual context, the self becomes the measure of all things. Any psychology that grows out of this context inevitably has an impoverished view of human life.

The problem with a purely spiritual approach, on the other hand, is that it sacrifices the outer life for the inner—it seeks heaven at the cost of the earth. The West is still reeling from centuries of repression inflicted by Christianity. Every major religion has cast a heavy weight of repression on the culture and psyches of its people. Guiding spiritual ideals become introjected as "shoulds," super-ego judgments that cripple emotional health. "Lower" or "negative" feelings, such as sexual attraction, anger, and sadness, become split off, and the body is devalued along with anything associated with it. In shutting down so much of the heart's feeling capacity, spiritual practice is crippled as well, for this diminishes the very feeling capacities needed to open the inner doors to the soul.

To maintain a connection to the heart, conventional religion has emphasized the higher emotional, imaginal level of the heart. The result is that much of conventional religion has become pietistic and effete, too highly refined, ineffective for real change, and unable to penetrate the inner veils that hide the true soul within. It is no accident that imagination, visualization, symbol, and imagery figure so prominently in the paths of the heart, for this is the language of the higher emotional part of our being. But too often practice becomes stuck here, satisfied with imagination or trapped in an inner fantasy world. Escape to heaven comes as a natural result, for changing human nature seems too difficult.

Many traditions try to remedy this disability by engaging the lower and central emotional energies through such things as singing, dancing, loud music, and rituals. Sometimes these practices can create inner openings to genuine spiritual states. But their disadvantage is that stirring up the emotional energies can produce a passionate froth and foam on the surface of consciousness that destroys the inward peace and calm so necessary for the inner journey. Even when an altered state results, the noise and the frenzy of vital excitement can kick up a lot of dust that obscures inner perception. The underlying intention of engaging the full emotional being is laudable, but the means are oftentimes inadequate.

Traditional religions have not yet discovered how to bridge daily life and love (bhakti). As a result, religion is a thing apart, operating both as a taming force on humanity's baser instincts and as a harmful force of repression that increases the power of the shadow to emerge in unconscious, destructive ways.

Is there a way to embrace both heaven and earth?

Although psychological and spiritual strategies *appear* to compete, actually each works to open up a different dimension of the heart. Each has essential knowledge of its own domain, but each is ill equipped when it ventures into the realm of the other. How can we integrate the wisdom of each to create an integral approach to opening the heart? Given the present state of the world, there may be no more pressing issue facing human evolution than this one.

INTEGRAL OPENING

In front is the heart of emotion that psychology has mapped. Opening *this* heart gives us access to the entire range of our feelings, in all of their intensities and complexities. Within and behind the heart chakra is the sacred heart, the soul or deep center that spirituality has mapped. Opening *this* heart opens a new dimension of consciousness. Like moving from two-dimensional Flatland to the world of three dimensions, our psychic center unveils an inner realm of joy, loving peace, and guiding light for our life. An integral approach to opening the heart must include both, for only in this do we awaken to the fullness of authentic being.

The authentic self is not incompatible with authentic spirituality; just the reverse, as they flow naturally out of each other. This was not previously possible because, up until this point, humanity did not have essential psychological knowledge of the self. Traditional religion has historically sought to excise the self, to cut free of earth to gain heaven. The full significance of the shadow side of the heart, the lower emotional-instinctual nature, the central emotional, and the body was not understood by religion. They seemed too unruly, too shut to the light, leading only outward rather than inward. But the advent of depth psychology changes this.[2]

What depth psychology shows us is that the biggest block to opening the inner heart is a closed outer heart. Psychology is invaluable for opening the outer heart but is lost when it tries to penetrate farther. Spiritual strategies work for unveiling the inner heart but are not notably effective at opening the outer heart. Both psychological and spiritual methods are right, as far as they go. The difficulty comes from applying the wrong method to the wrong part of our being.

Religion often seems like a world apart from ordinary living. Contemporary spiritual practice is moving toward a new way—approaching what seems far through what is near, finding spirit through everyday activities of living, loving, hurting, and fearing. For this we need to deconstruct and reconstruct the traditional path of the heart. Depth psychology allows us to see what is essential in these practices and to strip away the unnecessary superstition, dead ritual, and historical and cultural baggage that conceal their deeper truth.

Viewing psychotherapy as a process of opening the heart represents a fundamental revisioning of psychotherapy. Modern psychology has produced a more sophisticated understanding of the heart than we have ever had before. As depth psychology shows, the self is striving for love, for connection, for self-expression. What is needed is to align the authentic self with the true soul—then a harmonization of our inner and outer being will take place. As the psychic light illumines the outer self, our life transforms. We have a light within, a source of loving joy that uplifts all of our relationships and work, filling them with an intrinsic peace and a fullness of being.

Opening to this light is necessarily progressive, taking time and focus, but one thing is necessary—*aspiration*—aspiration for a deeper living, aspiration for Spirit. Aspiration is the upward flame that carries us toward our source and brings out the full force of our heart's deepest desire.

It may not seem immediately obvious how aspiration bridges the gap between our inner and surface hearts, and the rest of this book will try to make this clear. For now, suffice it to say that *aspiration is the call of the soul* in its upward evolution, and this aspiration for truth, goodness, love, and bliss grows ever stronger as the psychic center develops and matures. In the ego, this takes the form of desire, but beneath desire's unquiet push lies the soul's deeper aspiration.

This flame of aspiration is our highest light and inspiration, called Agni's fire in the Vedas. Aspiration, unlike love or bhakti, is present and available to everyone. It is not difficult to find. It is this turning within to our deeper aspiration, this lighting of the psychic fire in the heart, that is of crucial importance.

DOING PSYCHOTHERAPY AS OPENING THE HEART

Becoming and being a psychotherapist is a process of opening the heart. It is a long inner journey of exploring and working through innumerable tangles and blocks to our own feelings. And in bringing a spiritual aspiration to working as a therapist, it can become a practice of devotion and love.

Love is a word that is used with great trepidation in psychotherapy circles. This is understandable, given the litigious nature of today's society and the abuse of this word as a rationale for sexually exploiting clients. But it seems ironic that a field that tries to get to the heart of human experience should speak so seldom of this universal feeling so crucially important to everyone. Carl Rogers came closest to understanding the importance of love in healing in writing of the therapist's "unconditional positive regard" for the client as an essential ingredient in therapy, yet he too shied away from using the word.

Viewing the client as an expression of the Divine, as an embodiment of Christ (as Mother Teresa would do), as a form of Krishna or the divine spirit, allows us to open our heart in compassion and love. As the psychic center becomes more awake inside, there is a spontaneous, unconditional love for all beings, for nature, and for the unity of all existence. The more deeply we go into ourselves, the more this love emerges. To speak of loving our clients raises professional eyebrows in suspicion. Yet if we cannot love our clients, then why become a psychotherapist? This love can be experienced on an inner level and need not be expressed outwardly or verbally, yet this is the most powerful force for healing that any therapist can offer. And when a therapist can open up to this energy, psychotherapy can then become a path of devotion and love that opens the heart of the client as well as the therapist.

CONCLUSION

The heart is central to all living—the source of our actions, the key to our relationships, the gateway to our deepest identity. Fully opening the heart is both a psychological and spiritual process. What we are seeking is our authentic self, infused and guided by our deeper, evolving soul. To bring our life into alignment with this deeper center requires opening our heart on every level. Such integral fulfillment represents the coming evolutionary wave. Freud said at the beginning of the last century that dreams are the royal road to the unconscious. Today, with an expanded view of the psyche, we can say that *the heart is the royal road to the soul.*

Heart-centered psychotherapy can be a bhakti yoga for the 21st century that brings together our inner and outer hearts. In the path of transformation, an inner freedom that rests on an inner joy and love can only be a beginning, not the final goal. Joy and love and compassion also must suffuse our outer life and heart. The surface, psychological heart of vital emotion must transform to become a radiant center of love in the world, for only by such a shift can the world grow beyond its current adolescent stage of development.

Desire is the evolutionary ladder we climb until, reaching a certain height, desire transmutes into aspiration, and aspiration leads us to love and bhakti. Of course, aspiration is there all along underneath desire, the basis of desire. It is the inner gold that produces the gross lead of desire, but this is only barely perceptible at first. As the psychic center matures and affects a greater refinement of the instrumental nature, aspiration becomes more tangible. Psychotherapy must therefore focus on liberating desire and aspiration, liberating the fetters of the heart so it may feel freely and fully.

Psychotherapy and spirituality come together in the heart. The heart is a pathway to immensely greater depths and richness in our life and relationships as well as to an exalted center of delight within. When the psychic fire in the heart is lit, there is a steady stream of joy and love that can act as a balm to even the darkest, most painful outer circumstances that life gives us. Lighting this inner flame is the focus of the final chapter.

Chapter 8

Designing Psychotherapy for the Right Brain, the Left Brain, and the Soul

> Awake by your aspiration the psychic fire in the heart that burns steadily toward the Divine—that is the one way to liberate and fulfill the emotional nature.
>
> —Sri Aurobindo, *Letters on Yoga*

This book has been making the case throughout for a synthesis of psychology's many voices, for a vision of health that encompasses and exceeds what each specific school of therapy holds as optimal, and for an integration of methods to achieve this. It has further suggested an integration of psychology with spirituality, for only in this can the depth of the psyche be truly understood, as well as a joining of Western and Eastern psychologies' theories and practices. The body, the levels of the heart, the mind, and the inner being and soul are necessary for this more expanded perspective of psychology.

This chapter takes up these themes and places them in the context of current neuroscience. Recent discoveries in neurobiology and neuroscience have exciting correspondences to the planes and parts of our being detailed by integral psychology. Although there is no perfect fit in every detail, there is such close proximity that this knowledge provides yet another window into the larger view of psychology offered in this book. Some research directions have even started to extend the edge of materialistic science and touch the edges of the spiritual foundation of consciousness, which we will see has implications for psychotherapeutic technique.

149

As neuroscience has matured over the last few decades, it has begun to shed new light on some of the insights provided by depth psychotherapy about the nature of the mind, the self, emotion, memory, relationships, and development. A convergence of research in neurobiology, neuroscience, attachment theory, mother-infant research, and human development reinforces and clarifies many of the understandings of depth therapy. It has become increasingly clear, for example, that the earliest relationship experiences in the infant's family with its original attachment figures (mother and father especially) profoundly influence the developing brain of the infant. Secure attachment is highly correlated to peer acceptance, emotional resilience, leadership abilities, and enhanced immune function, whereas insecure attachment is highly correlated to greater vulnerability to psychopathology, problematic relationships, and reduced immune functioning (Stroufe, et al., 1990; Fonagy, 2001; Russek & Schwartz, 1994).

As the brain develops from infancy to adulthood, emotion is the central organizing process that shapes it toward coherence or incoherence, and interpersonal relationships are the primary way in which emotion is integrated and regulated by the developing mind (Siegel, 1999.) Affect, and the capacity to regulate it, plays a central role in neural development and behavior, that is, the ability of the person to self-regulate and self-soothe as well as to make use of relationships for the integration and regulation of emotional states.

While split-brain research has investigated since the 1970s the different ways the right and left hemispheres process information, only recently has this research focused on the different ways in which each hemisphere processes emotion. Thus for some time it has been known that the left hemisphere (which controls the right side of the body) is primarily verbal, rational, and logical and thinks in terms of cause-effect relationships. The right hemisphere, on the other hand, is more intuitive and visually and spatially oriented, and in seizing the whole rather than analyzing the parts it makes spontaneous leaps of insight in its mental processing. As it turns out, these inter-hemispheric differences also reflect the different ways in which each side of the brain processes emotion.

While some researchers interpret the data differently, there is strong evidence to show that the left hemisphere processes emotion in verbal, logical, and interpretive modes that construct a narrative to make sense of emotional experience. Because it needs language for symbolization, it comes on-line at a developmentally later time than the right hemisphere. The right hemisphere processes affect in terms of primary emotion, bodily sensed feelings, and relational context (Shore, 2003b.) Because it is dominant in the first three years of life (Chiron et al., 1997) due to its early maturing (Saugstad, 1998), it is crucially involved in the basic affect system (Gazzaniga, 1985) and in the modulation of primary emotions (Ross, Homan, & Buck, 1994). Thus when the left and right hemispheres operate in an integrated fashion, a coherent narrative emerges that reflects the bodily sensed, primary emotional experience of the person. When the left and right hemispheres are not integrated in their processing, however, the left brain weaves a story that may be logical but not coherent, since it lacks the right brain's contextual understanding and experience of primary emotion in the body (Siegel, 1999.)

Certain kinds of emotional wounding affect primarily left hemisphere development, while other kinds of emotional wounding affect primarily right hemisphere development (Beebe & Lachman, 1994.) Siegel (1999) gives the example of the avoidantly attached child's and the dismissing adult's communication pattern as a left hemisphere-dominated communication resulting from a dis-association between right and left brain processing.

Similarly, we can think of different therapeutic approaches as accessing either primarily left or right hemispheres for emotional processing. Traditional psychoanalysis, with its emphasis upon verbal expression and its minimizing of bodily states and somatically felt experience, may reflect a left hemisphere dominance in technique. Conversely, humanistic-existential approaches that favor bodily felt experience and primary emotion but downplay verbal representation and narrative processing reflect a right hemisphere preference in therapeutic action. What an integral approach to psychotherapy that integrates body-heart-mind-spirit aims to do, and what neuroscience seems to be suggesting, is a synthesis of emotional and somatic dimensions of experience, or in the language of neuroscience, a synthesis of left and right hemispheric modes of processing emotion. However, before embarking on such a synthesis, we need to consider an additional dimension: the soul or the spiritual dimension of consciousness.

HEART AND SOUL

Intriguing research has explored the effects of centering consciousness in the heart. Song, Schwartz, and Russek (1998) have reported that simply focusing on the heart area increases heart-brain synchronization, which in turn has a measurable effect on reducing stress levels, increasing immunity, and enhancing mental performance (Childre & Martin, 1999.) Researchers at the Institute of HeartMath have published a series of articles detailing how focusing on the heart while feeling a positive emotion such as appreciation, gratitude, or love results in a series of physiological changes correlated to lower stress levels (Childre & Martin, 1999). These changes include lower blood pressure and cortisol (a stress hormone) levels, increased DHEA and IgA (associated with increased immunity) levels, reduced activity of the sympathetic nervous system, and increased activity of the parasympathetic nervous system (associated with greater relaxation).

A number of studies also have found greater synchronization between heart and brain rhythms in such a state, and such heart-brain synchronization is correlated to greater intuition and creative problem solving. Conversely, there is a greater degree of incoherence between heart and brain rhythms during periods of stress or experiences of negative emotion, which partly explains why people do not think as clearly when stressed. However, it is not clear precisely what focusing on the heart area means, or which part of the heart is being focused on, for in integral psychology there are different levels of the heart: the physical heart, the passionate heart of emotion, the heart chakra, and the soul or psychic center, hidden in the "cave of the heart."

While the techniques from HeartMath can be useful as a temporary relief from stress, they suffer from the same limitations that many strictly behavioral techniques do, namely, they impose upon the person a different affect state rather than facilitate the emergence of an authentic, deeper level of feeling within.[1] Helpful as this might be in the short run, an integral working requires a more thoroughgoing resolution.

The psychic center or soul, as discussed earlier, is located deep in the heart, behind the heart chakra, on an inner plane. The psychic center communicates not so much by thought as by an essential feeling, according to Sri Aurobindo. Since the goal of integral psychotherapy is not only the integration and coherence of the outer self but the refinement and gradual psychicization of the self, the opening to the influence and guidance of our psychic center is essential. For this, two key conditions are most helpful: centering consciousness in the heart and an aspiration for the psychic opening.

Although Sri Aurobindo is clear that there is no shortcut to awakening the psychic being, he is equally clear that spiritual practice can accelerate the process considerably. Although many methods may be employed, and the spiritual literature from around the world abounds in numerous practices, Sri Aurobindo extracts the inner essence of many such practices and describes two essential elements. The first key condition is to center consciousness in the heart, not the physical heart or even the heart chakra but the psychic flame behind the heart chakra, in the middle of the chest close to the spine. The second condition is to focus on a feeling of aspiration for the true consciousness, aspiration for the Divine, and aspiration for the psychic center to awaken and take the lead, or else a feeling of bhakti, love, devotion, or surrender.

Aspiration plays a pivotal role in integral yoga, as it does in integral psychotherapy, but it is sharply differentiated from vital desire. The ego *desires*, but the soul *aspires*. Vital desire is an unquiet, demanding, and impatient urge that comes from the ego. Aspiration, on the other hand, is the call of the soul in its upward journey. Aspiration is quiet and nondemanding, and it accepts whatever the Divine gives. Aspiration can be ardent and intense, but it is fundamentally peaceful, an urge from the depths of our soul for the Divine and all things Divine: truth, beauty, goodness, love, gratitude, and devotion. Sri Aurobindo's distinction between vital desire and aspiration is critically important, for it illumines why so much of traditional spiritual practice is ineffective or only minimally effective because it bases itself on vital desire and creates a vital whirl that kicks up so much dust inwardly that it obscures the deeper light of the soul.

The practice often recommended by Sri Aurobindo is twofold. First, concentrate in the heart, not on the heart but *in* the heart (actually behind the heart chakra), as if physically located in this area. "The heart in this yoga should in fact be the main center of concentration . . ." (Aurobindo, 1971a, p. 780). Second, from this station in the heart, concentrate on a feeling or movement of aspiration (aspiration for the Divine, for the true consciousness), devotion, bhakti, or love, or surrender to the Divine. This feeling of aspiration (or love or surrender) then takes one more and more deeply within. As the intensity of the feeling increases, the inner doors open, and the psychic consciousness awakens naturally. "Aspiration, constant and sincere, and the will to turn to the Divine alone are the best means to bring forward the psychic" (Aurobindo, 1971a, p. 1100).

It will be seen that there is much in common with many Christian practices, the prayer of the heart, Hindu bhakti practices, devotion, love, and so on, but a crucial distinction is made in integral yoga. For these practices to be effective, these feelings are to be psychic rather than vital, for vital feelings only stir up the emotional being rather than calming and purifying it. To awaken the psychic center or soul, the means must be psychic. Vital means lead to vital results.

In integral psychotherapy, lighting the psychic flame in the heart is the goal. However, along with this, integral psychotherapy focuses on bringing greater coherence to the emotional-psychological self, and this requires a good deal of effort to work through the many levels of psychological, unconscious wounding that so afflict the heart of every human being. To bring awareness to the heart's depth of feeling and the vast array of lower, central, higher emotional, and psychic influences is the main focus of integral psychotherapy. In awakening our heart center or psychic being, the path for most lies in working through layer after layer of wounding and defense. A first step is focusing in the heart, which begins to open the inner doors.

HEART-CENTERED FOCUSING

The pioneering work of Eugene Gendlin to develop focusing over many years of exceptionally well-done psychotherapy research (1981, 1996) has shown how attending to our bodily sensed feelings is a central process behind psychotherapeutic change. While focusing is in the tradition of humanistic-existential approaches to psychotherapy, with its attention to the somatic realm of experiencing, it brings out what may be the key ingredient in all psychotherapy. In studying who changed in psychotherapy, Gendlin discovered that whether a therapist used free association, transference work, role-playing, cognitive therapy, imagery, dream work, or verbal techniques, the underlying process, the meta-technique behind all successful techniques, lies in psychotherapy's capacity to reveal the bodily felt sense to the client. In the language of neuroscience, Gendlin brings into sharp relief the importance of the right brain's awareness of primary emotion and bodily sensed feeling in order to construct a meaningful explanation (or coherent narrative) of emotional experience. Interestingly, Gendlin discovered that feelings are almost always sensed in the central part of the body or torso. This makes sense from the perspective of the subtle body in which the three chakras between the base of the spine and the throat are those involved in emotional processing, so the torso is the area where the physical body resonates most closely with the subtle body and the *chakras* responsible for emotion.

A limitation of focusing, which it has in common with almost all of Western psychotherapy, is its entire focus on the surface self and body, its lack of understanding of the inner being and spiritual foundation of consciousness. Further, it has only a cursory knowledge of the transference and the realm of the unconscious mapped out by psychoanalysis, and it tends to downplay the importance of verbalizing or left hemisphere processing. Nevertheless, despite these limitations, it is possible to utilize the key psychotherapeutic insights of focusing so that these can be integrated into a meditative approach to psychotherapy that includes both the surface self and the deeper psychic center or soul.

Integral psychotherapy highlights the currently unknown but secretly overarching principle of psychological life—namely, that our life is an expression of our deeper, evolving soul. The self or ego is what centralizes consciousness for this outer body-heart-mind organism, but as we saw in chapter 2, the self or ego is itself a surface reflection of the deeper psychic center. The action of the self both hides the psychic center or evolving soul as well as is an expression of it. To find our true center, we must go within, using the self as a passageway toward our deeper being. As feeling is the language of the soul, and the inner heart is its seat, opening ourselves to the depths of feeling and centering ourselves in our deepest heart is the royal road to our soul and psychic center.

What I have discovered is that by centering consciousness deep in the heart with an aspiration for the true consciousness, aspiration for our deeper self, aspiration for the heart's authentic guidance, it is possible to focus on the bodily felt sense from a deeper and wider perspective. This heart-centered focusing inclines consciousness toward its deeper roots, and from there it can perceive the somatically experienced emotional material more fully. Of course, not everyone can do this immediately or perfectly, but over time this aspiration taps into the yearning for authentic being that we all feel. For some clients there is a natural sensitivity to the inner heart's wisdom. For other clients this aspiration takes time to produce a result on the surface, though there may well be an action going on behind the veil. For still other clients this may stir an influence that is entirely unconscious, and the work stays primarily in the realm of bodily sensed feelings and traditional psychotherapy.

In centering in the heart and focusing on the bodily sensed emotion, the client is able to verbalize inner experience in an increasingly deep and perceptive way. This action engages both hemispheres of the brain—the right hemisphere's perception of primary emotion and body sensing and the left hemisphere's ability to weave a narrative that brings a greater capacity to witness, to understand, and to inhabit emotional reality. This integrates both sides of the brain as well as brings the soul and its powers to bear on healing and awakening. Any area can be the object of exploration: the client's past, the present outside life and relationships, or the transference. Any technique can be employed to further this exploration: imagery, body work, role-play, free association, dream work, creative expression—as long as the technique is grounded in and emerges out of the felt sense of the client.

To fully open the heart we must awaken and reinhabit the body, which psychoanalysis has not fully understood, and we must work through the deep and extensive wounds to the self and its relational world, which humanistic and existential psychologies have not fully understood, and we must open inwardly through aspiration and concentration the psychic center and evolving soul, which no Western psychology has understood.

A key factor in all of this is the therapist's consciousness. When the therapist can be centered in his or her psychic center, or at least have the aspiration for this, and when he or she has done a good deal of inner work toward it, then a psychic field is created that more easily allows the client to access these deeper levels. There is always the issue of the client's receptivity to the psychic influence, and of the particular chemistry between the client and therapist, for there are large variations in each of these. But even when there is a seeming lack of receptivity on the surface, there can be an influence working behind the conscious awareness. The therapist creates a psychic field which, through resonance, can help awaken and open the inner being of the client. This can deepen the traditional psychotherapeutic work being done, and it also can work toward the opening of the client's psychic center. Though a full opening may be rare in psychotherapy, a more realistic expectation is for integral psychotherapy to provide another stepping-stone for the client's evolving soul and to evoke a greater capacity to listen to the soul's voice.

THE FOURFOLD PRACTICE OF INTEGRAL PSYCHOTHERAPY

Integral psychology puts the process of developing our human potential into a cosmic context. Life is an evolutionary movement of divine consciousness manifesting more and more capacities through a human instrumentation. Life is good and meaningful, blissful in essence, a growing expansion of consciousness in a creative dance of delight. Our task is to align with this process, using life as a field for developing ourselves in every way, on every plane—physically, emotionally, mentally, and spiritually—to unfold our abilities to whatever degree we can.

An integral approach does not abandon the world to find spirit but rather seeks to embody spirit in the world. In integral psychotherapy this means a free and many-sided growth of our being, healing and transforming every level as we progressively awaken the psychic light and open to the soul's guidance and influence. The division of our being into body-heart-mind-spirit is extremely useful, for it provides an organizing framework for the levels of our human consciousness and allows us to focus our energy on developing each part, separately and together. As human evolution proceeds, the means for developing our outer being will progress as new advances are made. Psychotherapy has so much more at its disposal now than it did even 50 years ago, and there is no reason to think progress will stop anytime soon.

Awakening and Refining the Body

Any comprehensive psychology must take into account the immense importance of the body in our emotional life. To fully open the heart means to awaken the body. And an integral approach to the body must take into account the subtle body, for the subtle body is the foundation of the outer, gross body. In bringing consciousness to the body, we normally think of consciousness as "in" the body. But in integral psychology, it is the reverse, as the body is a manifestation of consciousness. See note 2 for an extended discussion of processes to awaken the body.[2]

Opening and Purifying the Heart

Most of traditional psychotherapy centers on working with the emotional level of the heart—on healing the emotional wounds, traumas, and defensive maneuvers that so impair the average human being. Whether approached through the mind, as in cognitive therapy, through the body, as in somatic approaches, or through the emotions directly, psychotherapy seeks to improve the emotional functioning of the client. Integral psychotherapy makes use of all of the traditional approaches of the various schools and strives for a higher level of functioning than envisioned by conventional psychology. Not only the healing of old wounds and working through of defenses but a larger opening and purification of the heart are essential in order to awaken the psychic center with its inherent joy, love, peace, and the light of its unerring guidance. As the soul or psychic center is deep within the heart chakra, the heart has a position of premier importance in integral psychotherapy, along with practices that help work through all of the unconscious defenses and obscurations to this inner light.

Expanding the capacity to feel is the underlying process, whether this takes the form of learning to tolerate greater ranges and intensities of feeling or to better regulate and contain emotional experience and not become overstimulated or understimulated. The ability to feel is so damaged and shrunken for most people today. Repression and disavowal are the norm, and the poverty of most relationships, the endemic fear and shame that so restrict our aliveness and vitality, has created a sick society and conflictful global culture that can only be transformed through individual effort. Integral psychotherapy sees consciousness work as the most radical form of social activism, for only through the evolution and transformation of individuals can collective consciousness rise.

The many techniques and practices of psychotherapy can be combined into an integral working—active techniques, creative techniques, verbal techniques, somatic techniques, imaginal techniques, cognitive techniques, altered state techniques, dream work techniques—and as psychology develops, new methods will be discovered and further integrations will occur.

What is crucial is having a vision large enough to encompass all dimensions of the heart, not restricted to the narrow view of a single school or taking one level of the heart for the whole. This means not only the lower emotional instinctual self, the central emotional relational self, and the higher emotional imaginal self but seeing how emotion arises out of somatic experiencing and including the embodied self as well as how thought is part of emotional experiencing in the mental self. The largeness of the authentic self, then, has all of these dimensions that have been fleshed out by traditional schools, but only in integrating them into a comprehensive whole can the fullness and richness of authenticity be appreciated.

As the authentic self comes progressively on-line, accompanied by truly intimate and authentic relationships, meaningful work, creative self-expression, greater coherence will become the dominant psychological experience, and a more powerfully intense and pure aspiration for the Divine becomes possible. In working through the shame-laden wounding, trauma, and defensive structures, aspiration becomes less narcissistic and self-aggrandizing. The psychodynamics of humility require a good deal of inner work with one's own narcissism if these energies are not to get hijacked by unconscious forces.[3] Including the bodily sensing and organismic power of primary feeling brings in a stronger force, a greater intensity of feeling necessary for inner deepening. Together these allow a refined, purified, and powerful aspiration to emerge. This aspiration for the psychic emergence and the true consciousness, this longing of the evolving soul for the Divine, this call of aspiration that rises from the depth of the soul—this is what lights the flame in the heart and opens the inner doors to our psychic center.

Quieting and Expanding the Mind

The importance of the mind in human experience can hardly be overstated, for in the evolutionary steps of matter, life, and mind, only in reaching mind does consciousness begin to know itself and achieve a beginning mastery of itself and the world. The goal in an integral psychotherapy is for the mind to function as clearly, logically, and freely as possible. Training the mind so that it can reach its highest potential is an important priority, so both hemispheres of the mind need to be developed. The aesthetic dimension of mind centered in right hemisphere processing needs encouragement and stimulation through beauty and creativity in all of its forms. The theoretic dimension of mind centered in left hemisphere processing is heavily emphasized in Western education, leading to clarity of thought and perception. Learning to become lifelong learners is a key goal of education. Curiosity and the joy of learning are natural states of mind, evident in young children before they are being subjected to the education factories of conventional education.

Aside from developing the mind's talents, an integral approach also seeks to quiet the incessant noise of the mind and to expand into its inner depths. There are many meditative methods for bringing more tranquility to the mind, but perhaps the most efficient is mindfulness practice. Simply bringing bare attention to our ongoing experience settles the mind's activities. Silent observation or witness consciousness is the one activity that does not stir up more dust and noise but brings silence through understanding and insight. As the mind calms down, it is able to look within and perceive its deeper source. Although the mind may be intelligent and well educated, in the earlier stages of evolution it is outward and absorbed in surface appearances. As evolution proceeds, the mind becomes more inward as it starts to free itself from its absorption in externalities and purely physical realities. Calming the mind is a prerequisite to looking within. As this occurs, the mind expands into its interior spaces.

Unveiling the Soul

Integral psychotherapy works to bring coherence to the authentic, surface self and to awaken the psychic center. The psychic center's self-existent bliss, peace, light, and love gradually permeate the surface nature. As the energy and influence of the psychic center infiltrate the self, the surface nature refines and becomes more responsive to the promptings of the inner soul. While the full unveiling of the soul and its coming to the front is a very long process, its influence in daily life is available to every sincere seeker.

In the initial stages its action is out of awareness. It is the influence of the psychic center that first turns someone toward higher things: meaning, beauty, love, truth, spirituality, and the inner world. Moving in this direction further develops the psychic being, and the person is brought into contact with people, teachings, and experiences that continue psychic development. As the psychic center matures, its influence grows stronger. The person is increasingly able to tune into and sense an inner source of guidance and wisdom. When the action is wrong or would be a mistake, a feeling of unease comes, whereas in making the correct choice there is a feeling in the heart of rightness and clarity. Misreading the psychic center's guidance is inevitable. The old nature asserts itself, and such misreading can further sharpen the ability to discern the psychic discrimination from the vital desires and preferences that rule the outer nature.

Opening of the heart and liberating the heart's power are essential to bring forth the psychic center. Traditional spiritual paths, ignorant of the complexities and power of the unconscious forces and defensive structures that have a firm grip on the surface self, have relied mainly on suppressive techniques to harness the power of the heart. Although liberative for a tiny few, this strategy has been psychologically crippling for many, which includes most people in the East and West.

However, with the insights and knowledge of Western psychology, we are now able to fashion a strategy that truly opens up, expands, intensifies, and frees the heart and clears away many of the obstacles to the heart's inner center. Instead of chaining down passions and feelings, bludgeoning them into submission, eradicating their beauty, and in the process sentencing our feeling life to a barren bleakness, a crippled, cold, constricted shadow of its true splendor and fullness, we can release these energies into life, enrich our existence, and bring forth a more psychologically and spiritually whole person. And as the heart's life comes under the influence of the soul, it transforms, uplifts, refines, and channels our life energies in ways that further our alignment with the Divine.

Mindfulness practice is the most direct route to the atman (Buddha-nature) as well as a powerful method to bring peace to the mind. It also is a very helpful preliminary practice for awakening the psychic center as it quiets the surface mind and brings more consciousness to the inner world. However, the main practices for opening the psychic being focus on centering in the heart. In taking our station deep in the heart and tuning into the psychic aspiration that is always present, this feeling grows and opens inward. Aspiration, or love, bhakti, devotion, surrender—these feelings come from the soul and lead to it in a call to the Divine for union. All spiritual methods that strengthen the spiritual aspiration are helpful in this journey toward our psychic center, for in the end everyone's path is unique, requiring each one to find his or her own way. However, the power of aspiration brings the help we need and in time leads into the inner chambers of the heart.

INTEGRAL PSYCHOTHERAPY

The question can now be asked: Is integral psychotherapy an organizing framework for all of psychology and psychotherapy, or is it a specific school of psychotherapy? The answer: It is both. It is an integrating framework for all therapeutic approaches and a unique therapeutic approach in itself.

As a meta-theory or organizing structure, it integrates all of conventional Western psychology within it as well as Eastern psychology and the world's spiritual systems. As a specific approach to psychotherapy, it provides for a wide and inclusive system in which each therapist can adopt the methods that resonate with his or her nature. Each therapist is drawn to those schools and techniques that focus on the levels of consciousness on which he or she is working in this particular lifetime. For example, a therapist working on developing the higher emotional levels of consciousness will gravitate toward systems such as Jungian psychology or psychosynthesis. A therapist who is working on embodiment will be drawn to working with the humanistic-existential therapies and body work. But what will unite all such therapeutic strategies is centering consciousness in the heart, in the psychic center, in the aspiration toward the Divine, or else resting in mindfulness and the aspiration toward the atman or Buddha-nature.

Integral psychotherapy begins from wholeness and moves toward ever-greater wholeness. It begins with the client's aspiration for a better life, for health, for authenticity, and for a truer, deeper self and consciousness. This aspiration is a surface expression of the psychic center's aspiration for a Divine living and its seeking for Divine wholeness, for spirit is wholeness itself.[4]

Ideally, an integral psychotherapist will be proficient and engaged in all levels of consciousness—somatic, all three levels of the emotional, cognitive—but this takes decades of training, and in practice people tend to cluster along the lines they themselves are working out in this life. The common ground lies in the goals: bringing coherence to the client's surface self and lighting the psychic fire in the heart, even though it may never be spoken of in the therapy. In the therapist centering in the heart and aspiring to awaken and bring forward the psychic center, a psychic field is generated that facilitates this process in the client.

Finding an inner source of joy and peace, love and light, and true guidance and discrimination profoundly changes the possibilities for psychology. The contribution of Eastern psychology is to show that this is not merely deluded fantasy; rather, it is the denial of this that is a mental construction which takes surface appearances for ultimate reality. The definition of mental health must include such psychic and spiritual qualities as wisdom, compassion, far less anxiety and greater peace, inner knowing and discernment, inherent joy not dependent on outer circumstances, gratitude and love, and the absence of loneliness—the more so as the Divine presence is consciously experienced. Our life is an evolutionary journey toward this, and our daily life and relationships are a field of experience to help us grow into this consciousness.

All therapeutic methods and techniques can be infused with the psychic aspiration. The psychic center aspires for the deeper truth of being, for wholeness, for the Divine, for bliss and love and peace. Integral psychotherapy is a movement toward these, working to bring greater coherence to the surface self so it can hold the power, love, and joy that emanate from within. Every technique, every school of therapy, can be integrated into the integral framework. Nothing is excluded.

Integral psychotherapy is a form of behavior change (or *karma* yoga), a practice of mindfulness (or *jnana* yoga), and a process of opening the heart (or *bhakti* yoga). It also is a form of body work (or *hatha* yoga). Further, it can be a process of working with the subtle energies of the body (kundalini yoga) as well as working with altered states of consciousness and the beings and forces of the intermediate plane (a form of shamanic work and/or guided imagery).

Integral psychotherpy can be summarized as being multi-dimensional, multi-perspectival, embodied, relational, and transformational. It is multi-dimensional since human consciousness has many dimensions or levels—physical, emotional, mental, inner, psychic, overhead, and spiritual planes of awareness. At this point in psychology's development, integral psychology is the only framework to adequately account for all these dinemsions of consciousness. It is multi-perspectival in its integration of contemporary academic and behavioral psychologies, psychoanalytic approaches, humanistic and existential psychologies, and Eastern and spiritual psychologies. It is embodied and relational by paying exquisite attention to inner experience in an interpersonal context. The therapist is, as mindfully as possible, creating a psychic field through aspiration and centering within, while attending to the client's experience. The client is paying attention to the feelings and subtle body senses evoked in the relationship—the relationship with the therapist, the relationship with his or her body, the relationship with parents, and the relationships with friends and lovers, as well as all outside relationships. It is a dyadic meditation. In its two transformations—psychological and psychic—integral psychotherapy brings about a better organization of the outer, fromtal self or ego through a new coherence of the authentic self on every level—mental, higher emotoinal, central emotional, lower emotoinal, and somatic. The psychic transformation brings about a refinement of this surface self so it is progressively psychicisized, spiritualized, guided and infused by the light of the soul within. At its farther reaches, psychotherapy becomes psychic therapy. It is a seeking for a greater consciousness, an aspiration to be united with our own highest self, which, in truth, is a portion of the Divine. In this way, integral psychotherapy is a form of prayer.

From an evolutionary perspective, the true and ultimate purpose of psychotherapy, as opposed to its current practical and compensatory purpose, is to help the emergence and growth of the psychic center while bringing greater coherence to the surface self. As the self becomes more integrated and stably coherent, an integral, soul-centered psychotherapy can bring out the clarity and light, the peace and delight of our true nature, so that it may suffuse our normal existence and gradually transform this life into a higher, nobler, more loving and joyous living.

Appendix A

The Philosophical Foundation of Integral Psychology

Integral psychology emerges from the integral yoga and integral philosophy of Sri Aurobindo. Aurobindo's major philosophical writings are contained primarily in his magnum opus *The Life Divine* as well as in *The Synthesis of Yoga* and *Essays on the Gita*. They articulate a richly textured and widely inclusive spiritual philosophy that unites the major streams of the world's spiritual traditions within an evolutionary context of Indian philosophy. The following is a very brief overview of integral philosophy.

> The teaching of Sri Aurobindo starts from that of the ancient sages of India that behind the appearances of the universe there is the Reality of a Being and Consciousness, a Self of all things, one and eternal. . . . [T]his One Being and Consciousness is involved here in matter. Evolution is the method by which it liberates itself. (Aurobindo, 1972b, p. 96)

Two fundamental approaches to the Divine have emerged over the last several thousand years of humanity's spiritual journey: the Personal Divine tradition of theism and the Impersonal Divine tradition of nontheism. The rich variety in the major world religions throughout the world today can be seen as so many exquisite variations on these two grand themes. Although some religious thinkers believe that each tradition is unique, from a wider perspective a common vision can be

165

discerned in which each religious tradition brings out some unique aspects of these themes and contributes some essential development to the overall vision, even as it situates this within the language and symbols of a particular cultural and historical period.

The nontheistic view of the Divine is of an infinite Impersonal consciousness, of which the world, and everything in it, is a manifestation. Hinduism calls this infinite consciousness Brahman, Taoism calls it the Tao, some forms of Buddhism refers to it as the Void. When this impersonal consciousness is described negatively, it is called *nirguna* Brahman in Hinduism, or Brahman without attributes or qualities. It is "*Neti, neti*," or, "Not this, not that," for it is beyond all verbal descriptions. Mahayana Buddhism calls it *shunyata* or emptiness. Taoism says, "The Tao that can be described is not the Tao."

When this ultimate spiritual reality is described positively, and always with the proviso that it can never be captured verbally, Hinduism calls this *saguna* Brahman, or Brahman with qualities or attributes. Brahman has infinite qualities such as light, peace, knowledge, power, love, and beauty, but the three overarching descriptors are *sat, chit,* and *ananda*, or existence, consciousness, and bliss. Brahman is a self-existent, infinite sea of pure consciousness that is eternally blissful. Buddhism does not venture into metaphysical descriptions but explains that the realization of Buddha-nature frees one from suffering and opens into an infinitely spacious consciousness of immense peace. In Taoism the Tao is without substance or form yet is the basis for all substance and form.

The goal of life in Shankara's *kevala advaita vedanta* is to seek liberation from the illusion of maya and to merge one's consciousness into the atman that is Brahman. Our spiritual nature is the *atman* or Self that is one with Brahman, just as the *atman* of everyone and everything else is equally the same Brahman, eternal and nonevolving. Enlightenment brings liberation from the separate ego and a merging of consciousness into the infinity of Brahman. Like a river flowing into the sea, no longer is there duality or even multiplicity: there is only the one Brahman.

In Buddhism the goal is similar, though put in different terms. The nature of life in the normal deluded state of the ego is *dukkha*, or suffering. Suffering arises from desire and attachment. In penetrating deeply into the true nature of ego, one wakes up (Buddha means "awakened one") and realizes he or she had been living in a dreamlike state of the separate self. The ego disappears into a vast, spacious emptiness from which all things arise. There is an immense state of peace and calm, and the mind's chatter ceases in an eternal silence. Liberation from the prison of ego brings not only a feeling of release and serenity but wisdom, as the fetters of desire no longer blind one's consciousness. One's true identity is revealed to be Buddha-nature, identity with the formless emptiness of Pure Awareness that is the All.

All of these traditions of the Impersonal Divine utilize the path of the mind, for mind reaches toward the impersonal. Mindfulness or awareness practices in one form or another predominate in the meditative approaches of nontheism, with heart-centered, devotion practices serving as preliminary first steps of purification.

Theism presents a very different picture of ultimate reality. In this view, the Divine is seen not only as pure Being but as *a* Being, with each person an individual soul, a spark or portion of this Divine Being that partakes of this divine reality. This personal Divine Being exists both with and without form. Without form, it is experienced as the Presence of an infinite Being.

When imaged with form, the many figures of God throughout the world show the myriad ways this infinite Being presents itself to humanity. In the West, this supreme Being has been imaged primarily in masculine terms. Although India is well known for its nontheistic tradition of *kevala advaita vedanta*, actually most of India is theistic, and in Indian theism this infinite Being is imaged equally as masculine and feminine. Many people mistakenly believe that India is polytheistic with its numerous gods and goddesses. But Hinduism is thoroughly nondual, viewing everything as expressions of the One, the gods and goddesses so many masks or personalities of this One Being. Vishnu, Shiva, and Brahma are three of the major masculine personalities. Shakti, Kali, Saraswati, Sita, Parvati, Lakshmi, Uma, and Durga are some of the feminine forms or powers of this supreme Divine Person.

What characterizes the theistic traditions is the reality of the individual soul, which is immortal, transcends birth and death, and, in Hinduism, reincarnates. The soul is not separate from God but is an expression and a portion of the Divine. But in growing up, each person develops a separate ego that believes itself to be independent and has no direct experience of God to show otherwise. The ordinary material life brings the person out into the world where the ego becomes entangled through the physical senses and desire with outer, sensory pleasures. In identifying with the body-heart-mind complex of the organism, the ego loses touch with its deeper soul identity and connection to the Divine. The result in Christian language is "fallenness," or in modern language, alienation, lack of meaning, an existential vacuum that is soon filled by loneliness, anxiety, despair, dread, and the myriad attempts to escape from these feelings.

The goal in theistic traditions is to reestablish our relationship to the Divine. Spiritual practice in Christianity, Judaism, Islam, and the theistic schools of Hinduism aims at bringing the soul back into conscious connection with the Divine, the source of all love, peace, and joy (the Christian notion of "salvation"). Theistic traditions rely on the path of the heart, for the heart strives toward personal connection and union. The means are spiritual practices such as purification, prayer, bhakti, devotion, love, service, and meditation, with mindfulness practices used as steps along the way. But most people are so lost in their distractions that they do not realize just how unhappy and lost they are. Hence, they never seriously consider anything else. Spiritual practice is often viewed as a giving up of the only worthwhile satisfactions that exist, which is hardly an appealing prospect for most people.

When a person does experience some form of spiritual awakening and begins to practice spiritual discipline, however, she or he gradually becomes purified of the density and coarseness of outward, materialistic living and becomes inwardly receptive to the Divine light, power, and bliss that comprise the intrinsic nature of spirit. The soul calls on the Divine, the Beloved, for union. When the soul begins to come into greater contact with the Divine, an inner radiance begins to manifest. As the soul emerges from the darkness and the Divine comes nearer, the soul blazes forth with unsurpassed joy, light, love, and "the peace that passeth all understanding."

FORMS OF NONDUALISM

The nontheistic traditions of the Impersonal Divine often refer to themselves as nondual traditions. However, this is misleading, for it implies that theism is dualistic, which it is not, although it can assume this form, especially in the popular mind. The highest spiritual experiences inevitably converge in the nondual, and Indian theism, mystical Christianity, mystical Judaism (Kabbalah), and mystical Islam (Sufism) are all nondual traditions. In Hinduism, this nondual reality (Brahman) is described as *sat-chit-ananda*. The central question is: What is the nature of this nondual reality? Is *sat-chit-ananda* an infinite impersonal consciousness or a supreme personal Being?

There has been on ongoing rivalry between these two profound visions of the Divine. Each of these views of the Divine strives for dominance, declaring itself the primary or higher truth and subordinating the other tradition to a lesser or lower status. This is clearly seen in mainstream Christianity, Judaism, and Islam, and in the bhakti traditions of India, which admit the experience of the Impersonal Divine but as a subsidiary or secondary spiritual reality. Similarly, Buddhism, Taoism, and *kevala advaita* are just as adamant in elevating their view of the Impersonal Divine to the highest level and dismissing the Personal Divine as secondary or even as illusory altogether.

One of the greatest achievements and most appealing features of Aurobindo's integral philosophy is his synthesis of these two views of the Divine. His spiritual realizations, first of nirvana and the Impersonal consciousness of *nirguna* Brahman and later of union with the Personal Divine Being or *saguna* Brahman, progressively led him to the experience of the Divine as both Personal and Impersonal equally. Aurobindo, who freely alternated between the pronouns he, she, and it when referring to the Divine, put it this way:

> The mind tends to put the personal and the impersonal in the face of each other as if they were two contraries, but the Supermind sees and realizes them as, at the lowest, complements and mutually fulfilling powers of the single Reality and, more characteristically, as interfused and inseparable and themselves that single Reality. The Person has his aspect of impersonality inseparable from himself without which he could not be what he is or could not be his whole self: the Impersonal is in its truth not a state of existence, a state of consciousness, a state of bliss, but a Being self-existent, conscious of self, full of his own self-existent bliss, bliss the very substance of his being—so, the one single illimitable Person, Purusha. (Aurobindo, 1973a, p. 65)

Integral psychology rests upon the integral philosophy and integral yoga of Aurobindo, who has been called India's greatest philosopher-sage. Integral philosophy is a vast synthesis of the many varieties of spiritual experience charted by the world's religious traditions and put into the framework of Vedanta.

MAJOR SCHOOLS OF INDIAN SPIRITUALITY

After a thorough examination of the cultures of the East and the West, it must be acknowledged that the West has excelled in its exploration and development of the outer, material world. It is not that the East has contributed nothing, but that its achievements pale in comparison to Western science and technology. Looking at the other side of the world's achievements, the East, and India in particular, has excelled in its exploration and development of the inner, spiritual world. Here again, it is not that the West's spiritual tradition amounts to nothing, but that India has made a far more thorough and extensive exploration of the inner science of consciousness than any other culture.

"India's genius for liberation," as Krishnamurti once characterized this country's vast spiritual power, has followed the spiritual impulse down a thousand different pathways, has traced out and pursued more lines of spiritual development, and has produced a greater abundance of spiritual literature than any other culture in the world. The ancient *rishis* who composed the Vedas, the Upanishads, and Hinduism's other sacred texts also had an enormous impact upon Indian culture, which even today is steeped in the many religious currents that have streamed forth from the Indian subcontinent.

This polarity between the Personal Divine and the Impersonal Divine has been worked out exhaustively along a number of different paths in Vedanta. Vedanta has been an extraordinarily dynamic and fluid spiritual teaching that has undergone tremendous development since its origins 1,000–3,000 years B.C.E. All of Vedanta is a spiritual search for the unitive consciousness of *sat-chit-ananda*, the nondual Brahman. The crux of the disagreements among the different schools of Vedanta centers on two crucial points: first, their conceptions of the nature of *sat-chit-ananda* and second, the relationship of *sat-chit-ananda* with the diversity of this manifest universe. Each school has its own conception of Brahman, and schools vary in their view of how real the world is and the nature of Brahman's relationship to it.

Kevala Advaita

In the ninth century C.E., during a period in India when Buddhism was popular, Hindu sage Shankara put forth his philosophy of *advaita Vedanta* (the Sanskrit *dvaita* means dual, and the prefix *a* means non, hence *advaita* = nondual). This teaching began a renaissance of Vedanta as it swept throughout India, almost eliminating Buddhism's influence and dominating Indian philosophy for several centuries afterward. So well known has *advaita Vedanta* become today that for many people in the West, *advaita* Vedanta is *the* Vedanta, even though it then became a minority view in India and remains so today.

Technically known as *kevala advaita* Vedanta, or unqualified non-dualism, Shankara propounded the view that only *nirguna* Brahman exists, or Brahman without qualities. The world is an illusion, an appearance that Shankara, in a much-quoted analogy, compared to mistaking a coiled rope for a snake. Although the mind believes it sees a snake, when it perceives more clearly it recognizes that the snake was imaginary and that it actually was a rope. Furthermore, there never was a snake; all that existed was the rope with an image of a snake super-imposed upon it.

There are two tiers of reality in *kevala advaita*, the real and the apparently real, also called the metaphysical reality and the pragmatic reality. Only *nirguna* Brahman, the metaphysical reality, exists. Although pragmatic reality appears real and is useful for getting around in the world, in the final analysis, according to Shankara, it is illusory. Pragmatic reality has a utility in that it serves as a kind of base camp for those attempting to climb the Mount Everest of *kevala advaita*. Hence, such things as belief in a personal god or religion accommodate the needs of people who cannot scale the heights of Everest immediately but need time to prepare at the base camp. But Shankara insists that to ascend to the metaphysical level as soon as possible is necessary for the true seeker, for the base camp of pragmatic reality is denied absolutely in the end. The featureless, attributeless Brahman alone exists.

The appearance of the world of diversity is due to *maya*, the mind's power of illusion. Illusion manifests this false appearance of a world due to the mind's attachment and desire for sensory pleasures. Spiritual practice serves to sever these attachments to the world and relation-ships. Work, family, relationships, and service to the world, all are distractions to be dispensed with as soon as possible. Knowledge, or *jnana*, is the path, the mind's discriminative power to pierce the illusion of a diverse world. When this occurs, one is liberated into an unmodified, infinite consciousness that alone is the Ultimate Reality.

It is hard to overstate the impact of Shankara's *kevala advaita* Vedanta upon India. Not only did it displace Buddhism, which originated in India, but it went even farther in its world-denying philosophy of *mayavada*. *Mayavada*, or illusionism, would have an overpowering effect upon the spiritual and cultural life of India for the next thousand years after Shankara. India's intellectual sophistication and refinement are hard to surpass, but many of India's best minds over the centuries became harnessed to the service of the inner spiritual life to the neglect of the outer world. Seeing the world as an illusion hardly inspires effort to improve it but, rather, to leave it behind. The ascetic renunciation became the spiritual ideal, for if the world is illusory, then the sooner one leaves this illusion the better. In later centuries other spiritual movements that were less world negating would come onto the Indian stage, but this fundamental push to escape from an illusory world gained a powerful momentum and had an enormous influence upon India's development.

Visistadvaita

The first serious challenge to Shankara's *kevala advaita* came from Ramanuja, who lived in the 11th and 12th centuries. Ramanuja was the first major spiritual teacher to provide a thorough and sophisticated philosophical basis for Indian theism, founding his vision firmly on the Vedic texts of the Upanishads, the Puranas, the Brahmanas, the *Bhagavad Gita*, and so on. Later theistic schools would borrow from Ramanuja's basic positions or modify them slightly, but it was he who first laid them out with brilliant intellectual clarity and rigor.

Ramanuja's doctrine of *visistadvaita* Vedanta, or qualified nondualism, holds that the world is ultimately real, the soul is ultimately real, God is ultimately real, and liberation is ultimately real. Instead of Brahman with no qualities, as in *kevala advaita* (unqualified nondualism), *visistadvaita* views Brahman as imbued with infinite auspicious qualities (hence, the term qualified nondualism or Brahman with qualities).

Brahman has countless qualities or attributes, including being the supreme Divine Person (Narayana), Beauty, Truth, Love, Harmony, and so on. It is a realistic theism that subordinates diversity to unity but does not eliminate diversity as Shankara's system does.

Ramanuja's extensive philosophical writings brought respect once again to Indian theism and the path of the heart, bhakti yoga. Before Ramanuja the weight of philosophy was accorded to *kevala advaita* and the spiritual path of *jnana* (the mind). Ramanuja provided a philosophical base upon which bhakti became the highest path and where *jnana* was put in the service of bhakti and became a subset of it. Ramanuja was a *Vaishnavite*, or devotee of Vishnu, in the form of Sri Krishna, an avatar or a Divine incarnation here on earth. Devotion, love, and surrender are the spiritual practices that bring the soul toward God (Vishnu, Naryana, Krishna, and Hari are synonymous with God), and God's grace finally liberates the soul. In *visistadvaita*, the liberated state is not identical to Brahman, as in *kevala advaita*, but the soul remains distinct, free from bondage, ignorance, and imperfection, in eternally blissful union with Brahman, a concept similar in many respects to Western theistic views of heaven.

Dvaitadvaita

Shortly after Ramanuja, Sri Nimbarka developed the system of *dvaitadvaita*, or duality in unity, also translated as dual nondualism. It is a variation on Ramanuja's qualified nondualism, in which the world and the individual soul also are fundamental realities. Both dualism and unity are real. As with all theistic traditions, devotion to a supreme personal God is the ideal. *Dvaitadvaita* also is a Vaishnava tradition utilizing the bhakti path.

Suddhadvaita

The founder of this theistic school of Vedanta, Sri Vallabha, called his school *suddhadvaita*, or pure nondualism. He criticized Shankara for not being nondual enough, that is, for using *maya* as a way to explain the world or the appearance of the world. Sri Vallabha argued that if *maya* was the reason we see a world, then either *maya* is a power within Brahman or it is outside of Brahman. If *maya* is a power of Brahman, then this means it is an attribute, making Brahman a qualified entity who is not without attributes. Attributeless impersonality will then have to be given up, and *kevala advaita* becomes like other systems of Vedanta. If *maya* is outside of Brahman, then dualism is the result, much like the *prakriti* and *purusha* dualism in Samkhya. Sri Vallabha argued that Shankara is "Samkhya in disguise."

For Sri Vallabha Brahman, *sat-chit-ananda* is truth unalloyed. There can be no touch of illusion or falsity in Brahman. *Maya*, therefore, is Brahman's real power, producing real effects and not just false appearances. The world is real, not an illusion. The world and individual souls are real and part of Brahman, with bhakti the way to liberation.

Advaya

Yet another variant of qualified nondualism is Sri Caitanya's school, which survives today as the International Krishna Consciousness movement. For Sri Caitanya *sat-chit-ananda* is Krishna, the one Supreme Reality. Krishna is the Absolute Person, as Krishna declares in the Bhagavad Gita, "I am the support of Brahman." The Divine Personality, clear and defined, is the core of Reality, with the impersonal and unmodified Brahman (*nirguna*) secondary, his peripheral brilliance or aura.

Dvaita

Sri Madhva, the founder of the Dvaita school of Vedanta, went the farthest in declaring the reality of the world. Ultimate Reality or Brahman has two aspects, Independent and Dependent. Hari (Krishna) is the Supreme Being in his Independent aspect. Individual souls, matter, and everything else are Dependent aspects of *sat-chit-ananda*. For Sri Madhva, the liberated state brings about eternal distinction from Hari, with no possibility of unification but rather a relationship of ceaseless, loving communion with Brahman, in knowledge and bliss. Here again bhakti and self-surrender are the means of self-realization.

Shaivism

Just as Vishnu has inspired numerous bhakti schools of Vedanta, Shiva is a favored figure of devotion and inspiration. Shaivism is popular in both northern and southern India, and it has an equally sophisticated philosophical basis on which to found the path of love and bhakti. Shaivism has a split within it that corresponds to the Personal and Impersonal schools of *advaita*. Northern Shaivism is similar to *kevala advaita* in its elevation of the impersonal consciousness of Shiva to the ultimate and an illusionist interpretation of the world. In southern Shaivism, on the other hand, Shiva is the one reality, but liberation consists of union with Shiva rather than dissolution. Existence is not merely an illusion but a product of the power (*shakti*) Shiva puts forth. In both cases, however, liberation comes through divine grace.

Tantra

Much of the West now knows of Tantra through the highly visible and well-marketed images of sacred sex, but this is only a small part of Tantric teachings. Tantra begins with the classic Indian idea of the One Consciousness that begins the manifestation by becoming two, Shiva and Shakti, two beings that in reality are one indivisible consciousness. Shiva, the male, maintains the function of pure consciousness, while Shakti, the female, is the executive power that manifests this world. The boundaries between Tantra and Shaivism are fairly permeable, and there is some degree of overlap and mutual influence as they share common ideas, terms, and literature. They tend to blend into each other, and in both, the supreme Divine Mother, Mahashakti, is the source of all power and energy, the creatrix of the universe.

This divine energy is present in human beings, coiled up and asleep as the kundalini shakti. When activated, it rises through the seven chakras or energy centers of the subtle body to produce dramatic changes in consciousness. Spiritual practice aims to awaken the kundalini either through the traditional right-hand path of purification, meditation, bhakti, visualization, yoga, and so on, or through the nontraditional left-hand path, which often involves usually forbidden behaviors such as drinking, eating meat, and sexual practices designed to stimulate the kundalini force. Opening and surrender to the Divine

Mother, through bhakti, devotion, meditation, and so on is a central feature of Tantra.

THE SYNTHESIS OF SRI AUROBINDO'S *PURNADVAITA*

The founders of these various Indian spiritual traditions all base their truth claims upon the very same sacred texts. They each interpret these texts differently according to their philosophies. In fact, the Vedas, the Upanishads, the Brahmanas, the Puranas, and the other sacred texts of India clearly uphold both a personal, theistic view of Brahman and an impersonal, attributeless view of Brahman.[1]

Aurobindo's integral philosophy and integral yoga comprehensively synthesize the different schools of Vedanta and Tantra. Technically called *purnadvaita* Vedanta (Chaudhuri, 1973), or integral nondualism, Aurobindo's own deepening spiritual realizations led him to a view of the Divine as both Personal and Impersonal, with infinite qualities and beyond all qualities, dynamic and static simultaneously. These are not either/or dichotomies but both/and totalities. Spiritual consciousness transcends dichotomous thinking and moves beyond to a widely inclusive state of simultaneity and wholeness. Mental thought is exclusive, and spiritual consciousness is inclusive.

Integral nondualism (or *purnaadvaita* Vedanta) posits Brahman as an infinitely auspicious Being who is the source of all qualities and powers and is multiplied infinitely in the world. All beings are reflections of this one Divine Person, and all creatures derive from this supreme dynamic Creatrix. The highest Brahman also is a supreme Impersonality, and the universal forces at work throughout nature reflect this impersonal power of creation. All of the schools of Indian (as well as Western) spirituality contain important truths. All have discovered an essential truth of the Divine. Yet all are partial expressions of this integral divine Truth.

Aurobindo's *purnadvaita* Vedanta achieves a new integration of the traditional systems of India. The philosophy of integral nondualism endorses the truth of each of these schools and reconciles their differences.

> In a realistic Advaita there is no need to regard the Saguna as
> a creation from the Nirguna or even secondary or subordinate

to it: both are equal aspects of one Reality, its position of silent status and rest and its position of action and dynamic force; a silence of eternal rest and peace supports an eternal action and movement. The one Reality, the Divine Being, is bound by neither, since it is in no way limited; it posseses both. There is no incompatibility between the two, as there is none between the many and the one, the sameness and the difference. (Aurobindo, 1971a, pp. 44–45)

From an integral perspective, the various systems of *advaita* are problematic due to their one-sidedness. Each system of *advaita* (and Tantra) stresses on one side or the other the Personal or Impersonal, form or emptiness, saguna or nirguna.

As the one Brahman multiplies itself endlessly to create this universe, duality first manifests, a duality, it should be noted, that is not *dualism*. Reflecting the polarized nature of existence, this is a duality that is always one, though two in appearance. Some examples of this include:

Brahman	Maya
Shiva	Shakti
Impersonal	Personal
Purusha	Prakriti
Ishwara	Shakti
Consciousness	Force
Static	Dynamic
Being	Becoming

In Taoism, this One is called Tao, and it differentiates into Yin and Yang, the two primordial principles of manifestation. As Hinduism and Taoism discovered long ago, we live in a digital universe.

Another key aspect of integral philosophy is its integration of the classical paths of yoga. *Jnana* yoga uses the process of mindfulness and the mind's power of discrimination as its lever to lift the person toward the Impersonal Divine, as in *kevala advaita* and Buddhism. *Bhakti* yoga uses the power of the heart through love, devotion, and surrender as its lever to lift the soul godward toward union, as in the Personal Divine traditions of Vaishnavism, Shaivism, and Tantrism, as well as Christianity. *Karma* yoga uses our will and physical being as its lever to seek the Divine through consecrating all of our actions to God and renouncing the fruit of the rewards of our actions so that we may align with the Divine purpose or Tao or Allah's will. In each of these specialized yogas, one part of our being becomes the lever or focus of our concentration. Body, heart, or mind is developed, and the rest of our being is left aside. In integral yoga, all of these classical yogas are taken up and integrated into a many-sided development of our entire being—body, heart, and mind together—in the spiritual quest.

Finally, the special place of the Divine Mother in integral yoga must be acknowledged. Integral yoga is both a comprehensive structure that integrates the traditional Vedantic, Tantric, Buddhist, and Taoist paths and its own spiritual tradition. Integral yoga is based on the yoga of surrender, surrender to the Divine in whatever form the aspirant chooses, but with particular reference to the Divine Mother. Aurobindo himself experienced the Personal Divine in the form of Krishna, as well as in the form of the Divine Mother.

> When the Ananda comes into you, it is the Divine who comes into you, just as when the Peace flows into you, it the Divine who is invading you, or when you are flooded with Light, it is the flood of the Divine himself that is around you. Of course, the Divine is something much more, many other things besides, and in them all a Presence, a Being, a Divine Person; for the Divine is Krishna, is Shiva, is the Supreme Mother. But through the Ananda you can perceive the Anandamaya Krishna, for the Ananda is the subtle body and being of Krishna; through the Peace you can perceive the Shantimaya Shiva; in the Light, in the delivering Knowledge, the Love, the fulfilling and uplifting Power you can meet the presence of the Divine Mother. (Aurobindo, 1971a, p. 173)

Although integral yoga affirms the experience of the Personal Divine in all forms and beyond form, the Tantric conception of Shiva and Shakti holds an eminent place, Shiva as Pure, Radiant Consciousness, and Shakti as the executive power creating and upholding the universe. Surrender to the Divine Mother through devotion (bhakti) and work (karma) allows the seeker to open up to the transforming power of the divine Force, which purifies and reveals the deeper spiritual reality within.

AN INTEGRATING FRAMEWORK FOR THE WORLD'S SPIRITUAL TRADITIONS

Western culture, which has grown out of the Judeo-Christian theistic tradition, has recently become enamored with the Impersonal Divine traditions of the East, especially Buddhism. Christianity and Buddhism are each remarkable systems for understanding the Personal and Impersonal dimensions of the Divine, but what is lacking is a unifying framework that can hold and honor each of these respective approaches to spirituality. From one perspective, all the religions of the world need each other to make a complete picture. Any single religion is incomplete, for it presents only a partial truth limited by certain cultural symbols and images, generally confined to a particular historical period or philosophical context. The larger picture presented by integration of all the world's religions is more complete than any religion standing alone.

The view of the Personal Divine from only Christianity or Islam or Judaism or Indian theism is a smaller picture than seeing all of these religions together as expressions of the One Divine Being. Similarly, Buddhism, Taoism, and *kevala advaita* Vedanta all express certain aspects of the impersonal truth. Taken together, they reveal a wider, vaster field of consciousness than any one single religion. The view of the Divine is greatly enriched by recognizing and integrating what each religious tradition has discovered. Anything less diminishes the fullness and integrality of the spiritual truth.[2]

The next phase of spiritual development throughout the world may well be not the creation of new religions but the deepening of current religions and their integration into a higher order and a more widely comprehending whole. Each religion can be viewed as a subset of the larger spiritual picture, and each tradition offers specialized methods of spiritual practice. This may foreshadow a global spirituality that is inclusive of the entire spectrum of the world's religions. But what is most crucial in putting them all together is an integrating framework.

Aurobindo's *purnadvaita* provides such a comprehensive framework. Integral nondualism can be a container and an integrating paradigm not only for the schools of Vedanta and Tantra but for the entire range of world spiritual traditions, for it holds together even systems that are usually thought of as mutually exclusive, such as Christianity and Buddhism, Judaism and Taoism, and Islam and *kevala advaita*. Although both sides of the Personal and Impersonal aspects of spirituality are present in most of the world's traditions, one side is given prominence, while the other side is minimized. Integral nondualism unites the central aspects of these systems into a comprehensive whole, as it appreciates their unique discoveries without devaluing the contributions of other traditions.

An Evolutionary Vision

One of the most original contributions of Aurobindo is his synthesis of the Western scientific discovery of evolution with the ancient Vedantic quest for spiritual realization. Traditional Indian thought had neglected the force of history in its cosmologies and philosophies. The present age (*kali yuga*) was thought to be a relapse from a prior perfection, a degeneration from a golden age of long ago. Aurobindo's Western-trained mind corrected this lack of developmental process and historicity in Indian philosophy and put the spiritual journey into an evolutionary context.

Aurobindo understood the tremendous implications of Western science's discovery of evolution, but he believed that Darwin's momentous discovery of the evolution of physical forms and species was only the surface of a far deeper process that is unfolding: the evolution of consciousness. It is this evolution of consciousness that is the most significant aspect of the evolutionary story, even though it is not visible on the surface to physical science. The universe is a vast manifestation of consciousness that is slowly moving from deep unconsciousness through partial consciousness toward full consciousness.

Brahman created this universe; indeed, this entire universe exists in Brahman and as Brahman cast into form. First there is an involution, in which the infinite, blissful consciousness that is Brahman manifests this material cosmos as what appears to be its opposite: physical matter that seems to be devoid of consciousness. But what looks to be inanimate, dead matter is in reality a dense form of consciousness in a deep slumber, an unconsciousness.

Consciousness is involved, veiled, asleep in matter, though secretly active. Over an immense duration of time, gradually this consciousness manifests as Life, the vital principle, which signals the first emergence of consciousness out of the unconscious slumber of matter. One-celled organisms and plants evolve into the initial bodies of vital consciousness. Then animals evolve as the next stage of evolution commences: the gradual emergence of Mind. But for animals, mind is entirely involved in the body and senses. Slowly, over hundreds of millions of years, mind manifests more and more completely, culminating in human beings, where mind at last emerges fully in its own right. Language and abstract thought allow human beings to disengage from the immersion in the senses to which animals are subjected and permit them to open up to a far greater range of mental consciousness.

These three steps of cosmic evolution—Matter, Life, Mind—are preparatory steps leading to a fourth, the full consciousness of Spirit, which Aurobindo called the Supramental, a perfect, spiritualized consciousness. In human beings, the level of mind has essentially been reached, though much of humanity is still struggling to fully develop the level of mind and to coordinate this with heart and body. Now that these first three evolutionary steps of Matter, Life (the Vital), and Mind have been established, the stage is set for the fourth, the Supramental, to establish itself more fully than has been done before.[3] The human body, heart, and mind have evolved, so that Brahman, out of its own plenitude of creative being, can manifest something new, a divine living in a material form.

Life and mind are actually involved in matter from the beginning. In nature, the process of evolution is unconscious and slow. But at a certain point evolution becomes conscious with the recognition of a greater spiritual reality. As a person enters a spiritual path, evolution becomes increasingly conscious and speeds up, moving straight toward the goal rather than wandering slowly and unconsciously with no clue as to life's purpose.

From this integral perspective, all existence, life, and evolution are fundamentally spiritual in nature, and the growth of consciousness is the central purpose and meaning of life. If this is granted, then far-reaching implications follow.

Implication 1: The Necessity of Reincarnation

The first implication is the need for a process by which consciousness can progress step-by-step toward ever-increasing fullness. Consciousness does not spring suddenly and fully into being or leap miraculously from an insect to an enlightened sage. It undergoes a systematic growth, a developmental process of ever-increasing power, amplitude, depth, and capacity. Since a gradual, incremental development of consciousness is occurring over great spans of time, this requires a number of different physical forms within which to evolve. From an evolutionary perspective, the problem with single-lifetime belief systems (such as current mainstream Christianity) is that the brief flicker of one lifetime simply cannot begin to exhaust all of the possibilities of evolution or provide enough raw material for the full development of consciousness.

Reincarnation is a widely held view of the afterlife, both today and throughout history. Reincarnation has been a part of most other cultures, including Western culture in previous historical epochs. When a materialist view of life is dethroned and replaced with a spiritual lens that sees a progressive unfolding of consciousness, reincarnation becomes a logical and practical necessity with birth and death as incidents or transitions in the soul's growth.

However, the popular notions about reincarnation contain so many myths that it is often hard to take seriously. The first myth that Aurobindo critiqued was the whimsical belief that if we are not good in this life then next lifetime we can be born as an ant or a cockroach. Tales of people reincarnating as animals, insects, and even trees and plants abound in traditional Hindu and Buddhist literature. But placing the growth of consciousness in the center of the picture rules out such beliefs as simply flights of fancy. Over great expanses of time, mind slowly emerges out of life. When the development of mind finally reaches the human level, it is not possible to suddenly and magically jump back to a prior level of consciousness such as a tree or a frog.

Another major myth relates to the understanding of karma. In Vedantic thought, karma is the law of cause and effect, similar to the Christian idea of what we sow we then reap. But in the popular imagination karma has become an automatic process of doing bad things and reaping bad results or doing good things and reaping good rewards. Good karma has come to be equated with being born rich, beautiful, healthy, and successful, whereas bad karma is equated to being sick, poor, and a failure.

In Aurobindo's view, however, karma is not a mechanical model with the divine as some heavenly accountant rewarding so-called good deeds with so much success and punishing so-called bad deeds with equal amounts of failure and pain. The growth of consciousness is the main issue, not merely the development of morality, especially the relative morality of a given culture or historical epoch. In the development of consciousness, mere outward success or failure and material gain or loss are but minor incidents in the soul's growth. Pleasure and pain have importance in consciousness evolution as an impetus for growth, for most often growth results from some degree of optimal frustration. Too much frustration, however, brings despair, but too little frustration brings stagnation.

This raises one of the hardest facts of embodied life: the function of suffering and pain. Indeed, suffering is the starting point for many religions. Buddha's First Noble Truth is "Life is suffering." Christianity affirms this life as, "a vale of tears." From an integral view of cosmic evolution, however, pain and suffering are a necessary part of the cosmic manifestation. Pain has an essential role in the soul's growth.

Pain and pleasure are two sides of the same sensational coin, both essential parts of the polarized nature of human consciousness. Duality and the opposites are facts of psychological experience. The spiritual task before us is to move beyond the opposites to a unifying perception of spirit within and behind everything. The divine leading is through the corridor of opposites: to unity through division and separation, to bliss through pain and pleasure, to love through fear and hate, to peace and silence through stress and disturbance, to truth and knowledge through falsehood and ignorance, to light out of darkness, to certitude out of doubt, to eternal life out of birth and death, and to consciousness out of the depths of unconsciousness.

The goal of life is growth, not pleasure. It is not that we should deny ourselves pleasure, but the "good life" from this spiritual perspective is a terrestrial adventure, a continual discovery of new abilities and powers, a development of consciousness and an expression of the soul's creative capacity to relate to the rest of creation in a play of love and delight, a bliss beyond pleasure. The pursuit of pleasure is only a first, crude approximation of this, and a single-minded focus on pleasure inescapably brings pain and stagnation in its wake.

To be born rich, for example, is very often a curse, for one of the main motivators to develop oneself is often lacking. More rare is the soul who is wise enough to use money not merely for self-indulgence but for self-development. It is not that pleasure is bad, for the capacity to appreciate pleasure is necessary for a balanced life. But when we look back on our own lives we can see how often our best moves came out of circumstances that were difficult or challenging.

Similarly, being born rich, attractive, and successful easily lulls a person to sleep through a lifetime, wasting the opportunities for growth provided by such an incarnation. Many mature souls intentionally incarnate into difficult, painful life circumstances for the purposes of spiritual evolution. Pain and failure serve to activate parts of our self and can bring forth great inner strength and potential. Even when it is overwhelming and the cause of outward collapse, a growth is occurring within that carries us through. Pain is a prod for growth. It opens up new possibilities of being, opens the heart to new levels of love and empathy, activates us to new levels of activity, and gives us feedback that certain life directions may be unhelpful or wrong. For it is the deeper soul that is evolving, though this growth may not be obvious on the surface. Each new lifetime presents the developing soul with the freedom to choose experiences that will support its growth or result in its stagnation.

Implication 2: The Universe Is Real, Not an Illusion

The second implication of an evolutionary view is that there *is* a point to creation. It is not just an illusion or a bad dream. Rather, this universe is a very real creation, a progressive spiritual manifestation leading to a greater divine life.

Mayavada, or the illusionist view of the world, has had an enormous influence on the East, much of it detrimental, and it is becoming more popular in the West as Eastern religion spreads. Is the universe merely a hallucination, a psychotic nightmare for which the only solution is to wake up as soon as possible and escape this manifest existence? To see life as an illusion, a figment of our imagination or a bad dream created by Brahman's power of *maya*, makes this universe seem like a stupendous waste of energy, thrown away on the creation of a cosmos that is basically of no use. Is the final result of the supreme and infinite wisdom of Brahman simply a gigantic waste of time, like some bad cosmic joke? Does this universe really amount to nothing?[4]

The illusionist explanation of the world (*mayavada*) that exalts escape from embodied existence is ultimately unsatisfactory from an integral perspective, for it avoids the very problem human beings are here to solve. Dismissing existence as a fantasy or dream cuts us off from life, whereas the evolutionary force of which we are an expression aims for a mastery of life. Instead, integral philosophy sees *maya* as the creative power of Brahman, utterly real, infinitely creative, a power of divine wisdom beyond the mind's ability to fathom. Integral yoga seeks not a release from life but a liberation into life, not a spiritual escape away from physical nature but a spiritual victory within our bodily existence.

Implication 3: Evolution Is Not Over

Evolution has not stopped. We human beings are not finished products but transitional creatures. Once a certain degree of physical, emotional, and mental development has occurred, we become ready for the spiritual transformation, the emergence of the next evolutionary step. Whereas the first long preparatory steps of evolution were to a large extent outward, making ready an instrumental nature, the next spiritual step is more inward.

If there is an ongoing destruction and creation of new bodies, new selves, then the question that naturally presents itself is: What is evolving? What is continuous in this process to experience a physical-emotional-mental-spiritual evolution? In integral yoga, it is the soul within that evolves.

The soul at first is a spark of the Divine in the manifestation that grows slowly into a flame. The soul extracts the spiritual essence of each lifetime and makes a soul growth from this experience. Gradually, through experience after experience, body after body, the soul develops an individuality, a soul personality, which Aurobindo calls the psychic being or psychic center. Because the language of "soul" is so contaminated by conflicting meanings, Aurobindo returned to the root meaning of psyche as soul to denote our deeper spiritual individuality, our true psychic center. The terms *soul, psychic being*, and *psychic center* refer to our spiritual individuality, a spiritual essence that grows from lifetime to lifetime, with each new cycle putting forth a new body-heart-mind instrument by which it develops.

The beginning human lives are almost entirely lost in sheer outwardness and density. But as the psychic center develops, gradually a greater light from within begins to guide the person. Instead of being led entirely by the body, the emotions, or the mind, a new guidance begins as the psychic center or soul illumines the way.

As the soul or psychic center comes forward, a palpable sense of joy and self-existent bliss becomes our normal experience. There comes a deep inner peace along with an inner intimacy and a loving connection to the world and the beings within it. We are led by a light within to express our unique contribution to the world's ongoing evolution. The path of the soul's terrestrial adventure becomes clear, the ego's confusions melt away, and we become increasingly conscious participants in life's great evolutionary adventure.

SUMMARY

Integral philosophy is a wide, integrative structure that holds within it the major streams of world spirituality. It sees the Divine as equally Personal and Impersonal and this universe as its creative expression. The evolution of consciousness is the hidden meaning of this material universe. It is a growth from unconsciousness to partial consciousness (in plants and animals) to self-consciousness (in humans) toward full consciousness.

The next evolutionary step is to fully embody spirit and bring a Divine living into this world. To bring the Light, Love, Bliss, Knowledge, and Peace of the Divine into this material plane is to transform it, to reshape it into "a heaven on earth." This means not abandoning the body and physical existence but participating in its creative, blissful unfolding, and for this the development of our spiritual individuality is essential. As human beings develop, we come to realize our deeper spiritual identity as both the growing soul and the unevolving atman. Awakening our psychic center or true soul and bringing it forward so that it will be a luminous guide in the evolutionary adventure of our life is the goal of integral yoga and integral psychology.

Appendix B

An Integral Approach to Spiritual Emergency

One of the most dramatic and fascinating ways that psychology and spirituality come together is in the phenomenon of spiritual emergency. This appendix brings the integral model to bear on the issue of spiritual emergency in the hopes of bringing some theoretical order and clarity to this puzzling experience.

For the vast majority of people, opening up to spiritual experience is a welcome and an easily integrated process. However, for a small minority, spiritual experience occurs so rapidly or forcefully that it becomes destabilizing, producing a psycho-spiritual crisis. This is where spiritual emergence becomes spiritual emergency.

All the world's spiritual traditions warn about different dangers along the way, the "perils of the path." New and expanded states of consciousness can overwhelm the ego. An infusion of powerful spiritual energies can flood the body and mind, fragmenting the structures of the self and temporarily incapacitating the person until they can be assimilated. With kundalini awakening, for example, there is an inrush of energies along the spine and throughout the body that can overwhelm and incapacitate the ego and leave the person adrift in a sea of profound consciousness changes at every level—physical, emotional, mental. Spiritual systems have identified numerous types of spiritual crises in which the ego's usual coping mechanisms are overcome.

Transpersonal psychology has shown how these crises are a kind of nonpathological developmental crisis that can have powerfully transformative effects on a person's life when supported and allowed to run their course to completion (Grof & Grof, 1989; Lukoff, 1998; Cortright, 1997; Perry, 1976). The idea of spiritual emergency has gained prominence in the last decade. It includes phenomena ranging from the opening up to psychic or paranormal abilities to the emergence of various kinds of altered states of consciousness.

Spiritual emergency was once dismissed by the psychiatric and psychotherapeutic establishment as merely a form of mental illness, requiring immediate medication and hospitalization in order to end it as soon as possible. This misdiagnosis and mistreatment aborted an otherwise growthful process of psycho-spiritual change. There have been numerous reported cases of individuals having their process frozen through medication and attendant psychiatric treatment. When the process becomes suspended like this, the individual is unable to complete the process and ends up feeling shamed and hurt by the misdiagnosis and mishandling, sometimes feeling doomed to having a lifelong mental illness that is actually but an artifact of this iatrogenic mistreatment.

Spiritual emergency is one area where the field of transpersonal psychology has had a significant impact on the larger field of psychology and psychiatry. The most recent edition of the Diagnostic and Statistical Manual of the American Psychiatric Association (DSM-IV), with the guidance of several transpersonally oriented psychologists and psychiatrists, now includes spiritual emergency as a diagnostic category under the classification "Spiritual or Religious Problem," a nonpathological V Code that may be a focus of treatment. This represents a considerable change in attitudes in the mental health community toward religion and spirituality.

However, despite this inclusion into the DSM-IV, there has been little impact upon clinical practice in terms of how the mental health field as a whole treats spiritual emergency. In part, this is due to the lack of training and education about this process in the mental health field and the confusion that exists about the phenomenon itself.

There are three major theoretical and clinical problems in this area. The first is the number and types of spiritual emergency. The current classificatory schemes are complex and cumbersome. The most widely used classification of spiritual emergency originated with the Grofs' book *Spiritual Emergency* (Grof & Grof, 1989), in which 10 categories of spiritual emergency are listed, including: shamanic crisis, the awakening of kundalini, episodes of unitive consciousness, psychological renewal through return to center (a particular form of psychosis), the crisis of psychic opening, past-life experiences, communications with spirit guides and "channeling," near-death experiences, encounters with UFOs, and possession states. These categories are phenomenological descriptions based on how people undergoing a spiritual emergency describe them; no claims are made for their objective validity.

Lukoff, Lu, and Turner (1998) list 23 categories of spiritual emergency, adding such things as loss of faith, joining or leaving a new religious movement or cult, questioning of spiritual values, meditation-related problems, and others that are concomitant with DSM-IV mental disorders. Nelson (1990) also includes Washburn's (1988) regression in the service of transcendence as another type, such as is often seen during the midlife crisis. Additional categories have been reported by others in the field. The Spiritual Emergence Network has identified "guru attack," the death and dying process, and addictions. The DSM-IV scheme for identifying such problems that are concurrent with other diagnostic categories makes for over 50 possible types.

These ways of organizing the field of spiritual emergency are clinically confusing and theoretically inconsistent. As it now stands, the category spiritual emergency is a jumble of dissimilar categories, ranging from the deepest psychotic process to the highest states of mystical realization. How can a clinically meaningful diagnostic classification emerge from such widely different levels of functioning? Is it possible to make sense of these very disparate phenomena? Is there a simpler way to organize this field that reflects a deeper order to this process? Can the whole phenomenon of spiritual emergency be organized into a coherent whole? That is the first task of this appendix.

A second problem confronting the clinician who is dealing with clients in various degrees of psycho-spiritual crisis is determining how best to intervene. What interventions can most effectively facilitate this process so it can develop optimally? For some types of spiritual emergency, certain interventions are indicated, while for others, the exact opposite is required. How can we best match intervention strategies with appropriate differential diagnoses? Suggesting meaningful treatment strategies is the second task.

A third problem is how to ascertain what is actually going on for a client. Depth psychology gives us a great appreciation of the psyche's capacity for fantasy, imagination, and self-deception. For many people, the self-diagnosis of a spiritual emergency is much more appealing than that of, for example, paranoid schizophrenia. What portion of these phenomena is a true spiritual infusion of higher energies and mystical states, what portion consists of images and fantasies from the collective unconscious, and what part is an eruption from the individual's personal unconscious?

A NEW WAY OF VIEWING SPIRITUAL EMERGENCY

Taking a simplified version of an integral schema of the psyche, various types of spiritual emergency can be viewed as being centered at a particular level of consciousness. This proves useful theoretically as a framework for organizing the entire field of spiritual emergency. It also proves clinically useful by providing a basis for assessment and devising intervention strategies to assist the process toward resolution.

It is important to recognize that there are no hard-and-fast boundaries between these levels of consciousness. Each level includes all that is above it but not below, and each level subtly shades into the next level in a mutual interpenetration along the edges.

Level 1: Conscious-Existential Level: This is the most superficial level of consciousness, our ordinary awareness of the self and the outer world.

Level 2: Personal Unconscious Level: Following Freud, this is the plane of consciousness that Western psychology has explored most thoroughly. Though psychoanalysis has made the most detailed study of this domain, the existential and humanistic psychology movements also have charted significant areas, such as the importance of the somatic domain, and have expanded our understanding of this level.

Level 3: Symbolic-Collective Unconscious Level: The unearthing of the collective unconscious was Carl Jung's great discovery. This level operates in images and symbols, and it is a dimension of consciousness shared by all human beings. It consists of the archetypes, universal forms, or configurations of psychic potential that shape the psyche and organize psychological experience. This level is a meeting ground between the universal forces and the human psyche, a bridge that links the cosmic with the personal, a realm where universal forces take human form.

Level 4: Intermediate Level: This is the realm of the inner (subtle) physical, inner vital, and inner mental planes that opens up to the larger, cosmic dimensions of the universe, beyond the physical creation. Philosopher Huston Smith (1976) notes in writing about the perennial philosophy that this intermediate level is a part of every major religious system in the world. It includes psychic phenomena such as ESP and clairvoyance. It is the domain of the spirit world that contains good and evil spirits (*devas*, or angels, and *asuras*, or demons), ghosts and recently deceased souls, and fairies or nature spirits. This level encompasses different planes of nonphysical manifestation (or different *bardos* in Tibetan), including blissful heaven realms (or *lokas* in Hinduism) and painful hell realms. It includes the shamanic world, which has both higher regions and lower regions into which the shaman journeys. The intermediate level also involves the subtle body or astral body as well as the energy of kundalini and the chakras or energy centers within the human energy field (the aura).

Level 5: Soul or Spirit Level: The central being is the ground of consciousness. Above it is atman or Buddha-nature, the eternal and nonevolving spirit that is one with the Divine and that part of us that is emphasized by the nontheistic systems such as Buddhism and *kevela advaita vedanta.* Below, here in the manifestation, it is the evolving soul or psychic center, our unique spiritual individuality, a spark of the Divine, that is highlighted by the theistic traditions of the world such as Christianity, Judaism, and Islam.

LEVELS OF CONSCIOUSNESS AND TYPES OF SPIRITUAL EMERGENCY

Locating different forms of spiritual emergency within different levels of consciousness yields a framework in which to organize the various phenomena into more easily understandable categories. Further, by gearing intervention strategies to specific levels of consciousness, this gives us a key for both assessment and treatment.

The conscious-existential level includes such kinds of spiritual emergency as a crisis of faith (either a loss of faith or a change of faith), conversion experiences that can be temporarily destabilizing, such as being "reborn," a change in denomination that leads some people into counseling, an existential crisis of meaning or questioning of values, joining a new religious movement, coming out of a cult, and separating from a spiritual teacher.

> Robert had spent eight years as a disciple of a teacher who emphasized surrender and obedience. After some time he had become one of the guru's attendants. During this time he loved the teacher very much and felt privileged to serve him, feeling that he was being transformed by his close proximity with such a highly evolved being. His departure from the teacher's spiritual community came in the aftermath of allegations of financial and sexual misconduct.
>
> Long before his departure, the guru had frequently embarrassed Robert publicly, humiliating him in front of large classes, castigating him for incompetence, and, on several occasions in private, beating him. Robert's response had not been to rebel, but to internalize his teacher's criticisms and to come back for more. He had held out the hope that by continuing to remain under the teacher's guidance he might yet win some great praise, confirmation, or sponsorship from his "mentor" that would enable him to advance spiritually. In the course of therapy, Robert began slowly and painfully to recognize how the abusiveness of this relationship was virtually a replica of his relationship with his father—an angry alcoholic who had humiliated and physically injured Robert, and whose approval Robert had always doggedly and unsuccessfully sought. (Bogart, 1992)

The personal unconscious level includes types of spiritual emergency such as what Jung referred to as "ego inflation" (or narcissistic grandiosity), dissociative experiences stemming from trauma or abuse, birth experiences, and any kind of delusional system or psychotic process that stays within the realm of the personal unconscious but that also has spiritual content.

> Tim had a long history of meditation, attempting to attain higher states of consciousness. Along the way he had had a number of spiritual experiences that led him to believe that he had reached a more advanced state and that he had a role as a teacher for the New Age. He was a remarkable individual in

many respects, highly intelligent, and he had gathered around him students interested in his blend of psychology and spirituality. Yet he had done little personal psychological work. Although not psychotic or delusional in his daily life, indeed, his professional functioning was at a high level, nevertheless his grandiose fantasies exposed his narcissistic character structure and caused him to limit his social life only to others who truly believed in him. He was able to maintain this stance for a number of years before his world finally began to fall apart. Initially believing his misfortunes were the result of demonic forces out to thwart his revelatory teachings, he soon was able to recognize and work with his primitive grandiosity stemming from his early wounding. (Cortright, private practice)

Types of spiritual emergency at the symbolic-collective unconscious level include certain kinds of psychosis, specifically what has been called by Jungian psychiatrist John Perry (1976) "renewal through return to center," involving an encounter with the archetypal forces of the psyche in a dramatic healing crisis (see the following case for an example). This also includes various nonpsychotic archetypal eruptions where the psyche is flooded by symbolic material and images, such as what Michael Washburn (1994) has referred to as regression in the service of transcendence that may occur in the midlife crisis.

At age 19, after returning home from hitchhiking in Mexico, Howard became convinced that he was on a "mental odyssey." To his family and friends, he began speaking in a highly metaphorical language (of archetypal symbols). For example, after returning from a simple afternoon hike, he announced to his parents that, "I have been through the bowels of Hell, climbed up and out, and wandered full circles in the wilderness. I have ascended through the Portals of Heaven where I established my rebirth in the earth itself and have now taken my rightful place in the Kingdom of Heaven."

The unusual actions and content of his speech led his family to commit him to a psychiatric ward, where he was diagnosed with acute schizophrenia. . . . After 2 months . . . his psychiatrist wanted to transfer him to a long-term facility for further treatment, but he refused to go and was discharged. He then immersed himself in archetypal symbols and literature as part of his healing over the following years, changing the course of his life dramatically. When interviewed 11 years after the episode for a case study, he maintained, "I have gained much from this experience. . . . From a state of existential nausea, my soul now knows itself as part of the cosmos. Each year brings an ever increasing sense of contentment. (Lukoff and Everest, 1985, pp. 123–153)

The intermediate level of spiritual emergency contains most of what is traditionally referred to in the transpersonal literature. It includes psychic opening, shamanic crisis, past-life experiences, communications with spirit guides and "channeling," possession states, UFO encounters, near-death experiences (NDEs), death experiences (DEs) and the dying process, out-of-body experiences (OBEs), altered states of consciousness, such as psychedelic work, guru attack, and the awakening of kundalini (which is the most widely reported spiritual emergency). All of these phenomena seem to originate from some portion of the intermediate plane of consciousness.

Terry's experience of kundalini energy was triggered by an intensive weekend workshop involving emotional release work. Several days after the workshop she experienced an explosion of energy throughout her body that signaled the awakening of kundalini. It moved throughout her body, up her spine and through her limbs. Accompanying this energetic flow were profound consciousness changes in which she felt opened up and expanded, yet at times left her terrified and unable to function. Although she knew about the kundalini phenomenon, this knowledge did not prevent her ego from being overpowered by the intensity of consciousness changes within her.

She was able to take a leave from work for several months and work with a therapist on an outpatient basis, and after three months was able to begin working again part time. Diet, energy work, modifying meditation practice, grounding exercises, deep therapeutic work on the emotional issues activated by the rising kundalini energies, journal writing, and mobilizing her support system were some of the things that helped in her process. After nine months, most all of the experiences had

faded, but she had radically reoriented her life during this time
to be more fully aligned with her spiritual path. (Cortright, private practice)

The soul or spirit level type of spiritual emergency entails episodes
of unitive consciousness. They may be of either the nontheistic or theistic variety. Although kundalini awakening may reach into this level
for brief periods, it is primarily centered in the intermediate level. The
experience of unity with soul or spirit may be overwhelming or shattering to the structures of the self and prevent normal functioning for a
period of time.

George had been a Zen student for several years when at the
end of a month-long meditation retreat he had an experience
of what he called "falling into the void." His separate ego
simply disappeared into a wide and vast consciousness. However, many of the reality functions of his ego were suspended as
well, leaving him unable to manage even ordinary activities
such as ordering a meal in a restaurant. Although for many
years he had been hoping for such an experience of "no mind,"
the reality of this great mental silence severely impaired his
functioning. The Zen teacheri at his retreat recommended
more intensive meditation practice, but this seemed only to
worsen his condition.

As he became more disorganized and unable to function,
he was evaluated by a psychiatrist at a local hospital, who recommended immediate hospitalization and medication. He
narrowly escaped being detained against his will and lived mar-
ginally for the next few months, avoiding contact with the outside world and spending much time alone. Slowly he returned
to more normal functioning, at which time he entered therapy
in an attempt to understand and assimilate his experience.
(Cortright, private practice)

GUIDELINES FOR TREATMENT

Some general treatment guidelines are common to all types of spiritual
emergency as well as more specific interventions geared to particular

types. The first and most important principle in the treatment of spiritual emergency is containment. Although establishing a container is fundamental in any kind of therapy, in dealing with a spiritual emergency it is even more crucial. Clients must be completely safe and feel supported to experience and express whatever inner states or impulses are flowing through them. At times this means providing an external structure that supports their process in the temporary absence of internal structure. A retreat setting, a friend's or family home, or even a hospital inpatient ward may be required in order to safely contain what is unfolding within, especially in the sometimes dramatic, early stages of the process. Later on, as the process smooths out, more traditional outpatient therapy can be resumed, although even here it may well be that meeting several times a week, and for more than an hour, is necessary for a period of time.

The second most important factor is the therapeutic alliance, establishing a human connection to the person in crisis. The therapist acts as ground control, a stabilizing presence whose calmness and guidance during this turbulent time can be profoundly reassuring. The consciousness of the therapist is of paramount importance. The therapist needs to be impeccably authentic, not feigning more knowledge or confidence than is truly there, for in the heightened consciousness of the person undergoing spiritual emergency, there is an enhanced energetic and telepathic sensitivity that immediately picks up any falsity or phoniness that can jeopardize the integrity of the relationship. The therapist lets the person know that he or she is not alone, and this in itself can be profoundly helpful. The therapist should be trained in spiritual emergency as well as in psychopathology and be able to tell the difference between the two (as well as the gray areas where both are occurring).

Often the most powerful intervention in treating clients undergoing some form of spiritual emergency is education. Providing a psychospiritual framework for understanding what the client is experiencing gives the person and those around him or her a cognitive grasp of what is happening. It also depathologizes the process and can greatly reduce the fear and anxiety that accompany a misdiagnosis of psychosis. Education allows the person to go with the experience, to flow with the process and trust it rather than trying to resist or control it, which is the instinctive tendency when the experience is interpreted as pathological.

The therapist must bring an unshakable trust in the process to allow it to unfold optimally. Experiential therapy can be helpful in moving through stuck areas, yet equally important is the need to monitor how assimilable the experience is. The therapist must constantly monitor the client's ability to make use of what is occurring and maintain the delicate balance between opening and closing to ensure optimal integration of the experience.

Additionally, specific treatment modalities are appropriate for a given level of consciousness and the type of spiritual emergency.

For spiritual emergencies on the first level of the conscious-existential plane, therapy for crises of faith may consist of support for the person and a therapeutic dialogue along the lines of existential therapy, exploring the nature of meaning, values, and faith within the client's life. It is important not to reduce these existential conflicts to earlier psychodynamic events from childhood, though they may resonate with earlier developmental levels, but to engage the client at the level of meaning and the feelings of loss, insecurity, and disruption when this meaning is questioned. When the crisis stems from coming out of a cult or separating from a spiritual teacher, saying good-by and grieving the lost community is essential to moving on, as is establishing a new support system and finding new ways of meeting the selfobject needs that have been disrupted, as a traditional approach to therapy would advocate. Therapy with spiritual emergency at this level is similar to traditional psychotherapy and includes an existential and spiritual focus.

For spiritual emergencies at the second level of the personal unconscious, traditional psychotherapeutic techniques are again important. It may well be a genuine spiritual experience that has stimulated the grandiosity of the person. It may even be that the person still has occasional contact with a larger plane of spiritual experience that reinforces this grandiosity. Nevertheless, the central psychological feature of the presenting picture can still be organized at the level of the personal unconscious. Medication may even be indicated. Levels 1 and 2 are the levels for which traditional psychotherapy has been designed.

For spiritual emergencies at the third level of the symbolic-collective unconscious, Jungian and psychosynthesis techniques for working with symbols, imagery, and imagination are helpful. Artwork and expressive arts techniques, active imagination, and imagery are particularly appropriate. If the crisis is renewal through return to center, this involves fully letting go into the psyche's destruction and rebirth process, working with this process as outlined by John Perry's (1953, 1976) work and R. D. Laing's (1965, 1967) work as closely as possible. The tremendous psychic upheaval needs containment and support, which usually entails a well-staffed retreat or hospital-like environment.

Because there is only one word for psychosis, all psychoses are generally treated alike by the mental health establishment: drugs and hospitalization are used to end it as soon as possible. However, this view of spiritual emergence demands a discrimination among the different forms of psychotic process. There is a spectrum of psychoses, ranging from regressive, malignant psychosis at one end that needs standard treatment to temporary destabilizing crises such as bipolar disorders that may open into genuine spiritual states, especially during the manic part of the cycle, to genuine healing crises that need to be gone through and supported in the manner of Perry and Laing. Bipolar disorders should be ended as soon as possible through medication, for there is little redeeming value in the crash and burn that follows mania, whereas the psychotic healing crisis of return to center demands going with and through the entire process from beginning to end in order for full integration to occur.

One reason for discriminating among the different types of psychotic process is frequency. If this is the first or one of the first psychotic breaks, then there is a much greater chance of a permanently healthy outcome if handled skillfully. On the other hand, if this has been a pattern over many years or decades, then the neural pathways seem to become strengthened and reinforced, making a full recovery much less likely.

Spiritual emergencies on the fourth level of the intermediate plane require grounding, above all else, for crises at this plane of consciousness almost always involve the client being disconnected or detached from his or her body. Grounding is important at every level, but in crises at the intermediate level the client may go farther from the body into the subtle body or out of the body entirely, or consciousness may move into realms that seem to have almost no connection to the body. Grounding usually is used in two senses: first, achieving a more cohesive, integrated presence that can act in a unified way, not fragmented or flying apart in all directions but able to act in this earth plane at all levels, physical, vital, mental, and spiritual; second, grounding means coming back into the physical vehicle. Aurobindo's spiritual collaborator, the Mother, once wrote that the best protection against the hostile forces of the intermediate plane is the body. There are many different techniques for grounding, including such things as diet, exercise, bodywork, affirming boundaries, and even medication when used conservatively (see the final section of this appendix and Cortright, 1997, for an expanded discussion of grounding).

The treatment focus is on containing and modulating the intensity of the experience so it can be assimilated by the person. Surrender to the process is important but so is modulating the force and power of the experience so it no longer overwhelms the person's integrative capacities. Stopping, reducing, or at least changing meditation practice is almost always advised at this level.

Crises at the fifth and deepest level of the soul or spirit, on the other hand, involve surrender to the larger process. This allows the person to be acted on directly by the spiritual power at work, which is necessary for the internal adjustments to take place. This involves trust in the higher power at work and a protection and caring for the individual while this power is active. Ramana Maharshi had to be literally fed by hand for several months before his process stabilized, and he went on to become one of the greatest of all Hindu sages. The guidance of an advanced spiritual teacher from the client's tradition who can work with the therapist is helpful, although oftentimes spiritual emergency occurs outside of any tradition or may involve experiences not explained within a given tradition. Generally consciousness needs time to adapt to an expanded state, and outside support may be essential during this period of transition.

PROBLEMS IN ASSESSMENT

With any inner experience it is difficult to ascertain what is truly going on. When psychology was simply pure psychology, devoid of any spiritual content, the problem was much easier, because everything was seen as a product of the person's own mind. However, when transpersonal psychology opens the Pandora's box of spiritual experience, although it immeasurably enriches our view of the psyche, it also lets in some complex and perplexing epistemological questions.

For example, according to this map, true possession states would be considered level 4 or intermediate plane phenomena, but the experience of possession may occur on more superficial levels as well. That is, there may be personal unconscious level possession states that are simply a product of the psychotic process, that is, the result of the patient's own personal unconscious, where she or he feels "possessed" but is simply overcome by the forces of the personal unconscious, such as impulses from the id. There also may be level 3, the symbolic-collective unconscious plane, possession states that involve possession by a particular archetypal form, such as we see in Perry's "return to center." This is further complicated by the possibility that some possession states may involve *both* a psychotic process *and* a genuine possessing entity from the intermediate zone. It may well be the case that possession states do not occur with psychologically healthy individuals and always involve a person with a serious degree of psychological disturbance and loss of boundaries, and this may be what allows the possessing entity access to an unprotected mind. Possession that is the result of channeling is a different matter, however, for here the boundaries of the person are let down voluntarily, and the entity is invited in.

UFO phenomena present the same difficulty. Although people who experience UFO encounters view the experience as something that occurred "outside" of them (that is, as something that could be videotaped or seen by others), such experiences are here conceptualized as inner experiences. If this is so, then UFO encounters may simply be an opening into level 4, the intermediate plane of consciousness, interpreting such experiences in a more culturally recognized symbol system, that is, as aliens. Alternately, the experience of aliens may be an archetypal eruption from the level of the collective unconscious (level 3) or a delusion stemming from the level of the personal unconscious (level 2).

What is "actually" going on? At present, we are unable to say. It may vary from person to person, and even with the same person it may vary over time. It may even be a mixture of something vaguely experienced at one level (e.g., intermediate) and elaborated on by another level (e.g., personal unconscious) and interpreted by still another level (e.g., conscious-existential).

Another problematic area is the kundalini phenomenon. Kundalini awakening is the most widely reported form of spiritual emergency. However, the criteria for kundalini awakening are very broad and include powerful energetic states of all kinds. Sometimes kundalini awakening either becomes, or was all along, mania (bipolar disorder), anxiety states, and panic states. Whether mania and other high arousal states are fully or partly a result of kundalini awakening gone awry or whether such states are conflated due to similarities between high energy states remains an open question.

These difficulties in assessment have implications for treatment. In calibrating treatments to specific levels, the effectiveness of a particular treatment can help determine more accurately what is occurring and from where it originates. However, treatment strategies at one level, although usually most effective at that level, also may be effective for other levels. For example, the use of anti-psychotic medication can ground the psyche so powerfully that it effectively eliminates the experience of being "possessed," whether this possession is a product of the personal unconscious, the symbolic-collective unconscious, or the intermediate plane. As we learn more about these phenomena, more focused interventions may emerge that will help clarify what is occurring.

This integral approach to a depth map of consciousness greatly enlarges the picture of psychology. In this view, human consciousness extends to include cosmic, universal dimensions and opens inwardly to reveal the roots of consciousness in an ultimately spiritual ground of being. On this journey toward full self-knowledge, spiritual experiences can emerge in ways that disturb the balance of the outer, egoic self. To shut off this deeper knowing through medication and pathologizing is to tragically cut off a process of self-discovery. But when spiritual emergency can be turned into spiritual emergence, then this process can be seen as a rite of passage into deeper being, a developmental crisis that leaves both the person and the therapist with a deeper sense of the possibilities for healing, growth, and transformation.

AN INTEGRAL APPROACH TO INTEGRATION AND GROUNDING

Treatment of spiritual emergency must monitor the intensity of the experience to ensure that it matches the integrative capacities of the client. The intensity can be increased or decreased.

1. *Increase intensity.* This is widely practiced and has been the primary method reported in most of the spiritual emergency literature. Experiential therapy, such as deep breathing

methods, is used to facilitate the energies of spiritual emergency to move past their stuck areas and overwhelm the blocks that impede the experience. This can help move the process toward conclusion. When previous psychiatric treatment has frozen the process through medication, a common situation, this makes a good deal of sense. However, for many people increasing the intensity is not helpful, in fact, it only perpetuates or even exacerbates the crisis.

2. *Decrease intensity.* When the capacity of the client to assimilate the experience of spiritual emergency is being overwhelmed, decreasing its intensity may be necessary. The goal is to modulate the force of the psychic energies, to tame the disruptive power so it is no longer shattering. Slowing it down allows it to become integrated. Care must be taken not to overdo this so much that it stops but, rather, to slow down the process so it is gentler and less disorienting. This brings the psyche's natural integrative functions back into line so the experience can move toward resolution. Toward this end, a continuum of grounding strategies may be helpful.

An integral approach to grounding involves practices for the levels of body, heart, mind, and spirit.

The Physical Level: The following practices are helpful for reconnecting consciousness to the body:

Diet: Eat heavy foods, especially those high in protein and fat or complex carbohydrates, for example, whole grains, beans, dairy, meat or fish (if eaten), and cooked vegetables. It is best to avoid raw fruit and vegetables, simple carbohydrates such as sugar and refined foods, and stimulants like caffeine or chocolate. Think pizza.

Exercise: This is a very individual matter, for many people in the throes of spiritual emergency are not ready to exercise. But if the person is able to, she or he should be encouraged to engage in whatever physical movement feels right, including walking (in nature rather than on busy streets), running, yoga, and any type of physical work, such as gardening (all contact with the earth can help). Even such physical activities as sweeping, washing dishes, and raking leaves can be beneficial.

Sleep is very grounding and restorative. Generally the more sleep, the better, particularly when the lack of sleep is a precipitating factor as it often is.

Contact with nature in any form is encouraged. Nature walks, cloud gazing, outdoor work, and fresh air are helpful.

Bodywork can be helpful, including light massage, acupressure, or acupuncture.

Medication: Indications for medication are primarily a person's inability to sleep or the desire to take the edge off of a crisis state. It is best to take a minimalist approach, for overmedicating is the biggest danger in a genuine spiritual emergency. Many supplements and drugs are available, ranging from very mild to very strong.

> Calcium is a natural muscle relaxant. Taking an extra 1,000 mg in the morning and evening can provide a very mild, relaxing effect.

> Bach Flower remedies and homeopathic remedies are useful for anxiety and insomnia.

> GABA (gamma-aminobutyric acid) is a nutritional supplement that has a relaxing and sleep-promoting effect. Also 5–HTP, a precursor of serotonin, and the amino acid L-theanine can produce relaxation without a drugged feeling.

> Herbs such as spearmint and chamomile in tea form are mildly relaxing. Somewhat stronger is passionflower (calming without being sedating). Kava, hops, and skullcap are more potent herbs. Stronger still is valerian, which promotes sleep and can serve as a kind of tranquilizer.

> Alcohol in the form of an occasional glass or two of wine can provide needed relief to take the edge off. If the client has a history of substance abuse, then this should be suggested cautiously, for there can be a pull toward oblivion rather than simply a slowing down of the process.

> Tranquilizers such as Xanax, Ativan, Valium, Librium, and Clonapin may be used. For tranquilizers and the following two classes of medication, it is important to work with a physician or psychiatrist to prescribe and monitor these medications:
> 1. Sedatives, such as barbiturates, can be used.
> 2. Major tranquilizers (such as Thorazine), mood stabilizers (such as lithuim, Tegnatol, Depacote), and anti-psychotic medication (such as Risperdol and Zipexa), when judiciously used, can sometimes help avoid hospitalization.

The Emotional Level: Feeling connected to other people is emotionally grounding. In states of distress, and especially in a spiritual emergency, establishing contact with a therapist or guide is enormously relieving. The importance of having someone who serves as ground control and is a soothing, calm presence cannot be overstated. One of the most difficult aspects of spiritual emergency can be feeling isolated and alone. A therapeutic relationship helps counter this. Sharing the experience with a caring, sensitive guide brings a level of concreteness to the experience. It can be important to activate the support system of the person undergoing spiritual emergency, though this needs to be done carefully, educating friends and family so that they do not become fearful. When done skillfully, mobilizing the selfobject matrix of the person and reestablishing contact with important friends and family will extend emotional grounding.

The Mental Level: Learning about the type of spiritual emergency through reading is mentally grounding. Cognitively understanding what is occurring helps one get a handle on the experience. Verbal expression, through talking and writing, also is a way of giving form to inner experiences. Verbalizing, whether in a journal or talking to others, helps integrate the experience. However, it should be recognized that talking too much should be avoided and can even dissipate the experience prematurely.

The Spiritual Level: Very often spiritual emergency occurs as a result of stress, especially spiritual stress, which may happen during a meditation retreat. Stopping, changing, or decreasing meditation is almost always advised when the experience gets out of hand. Each person needs to experiment to see what intensifies the experience and what helps modulate it. Certain meditative practices can be helpful in this regard.

Conventional wisdom in transpersonal circles has it that mindfulness practice opens up the person and should be avoided here, while concentration practices are grounding and encouraged. However, clinical experience proves this to be a facile distinction that may not be helpful. This is such an individual affair and depends on the person, the context, the background of the person, and other factors. In practice, mindfulness practices may strengthen the inner being and help develop a witness consciousness that helps navigate this experience. And in concentrations, practices the person may pour his or her consciousness into the object of concentration and actually intensify the overwhelming qualities of the experience. It is a far more complex matter than this distinction implies. The following practices have been shown to be helpful at times:

1. Prayer and focus on the Divine: This is useful especially if the person is open to a theistic path. Even if the person is a Buddhist, invoking the help of a Boddhisattva can be reassuring.
2. Breath meditation: By making the physical sensations of breathing the object of meditative focus, Buddhist meditation on the breath has the wonderful effect of bringing consciousness into the body and also is profoundly relaxing and anxiety reducing.
3. Mantra: A great deal of current research shows that the repetition of a mantra produces calmness and physical relaxation for most people. However, in the field of spiritual emergency, there is less data on the effects of mantra. Mantra is a complex phenomenon, and physical relaxation is only one of its effects. Clinical experience demonstrates that many people experience an opening to an inner plane that leaves them feeling more spacey and less grounded in the body, and for these people mantra may be contraindicated. For others, however, this a perfectly fine and helpful practice.
4. Concentration on an object: This practice, such as concentrating on a flower or candle or sound such as music, can steady the consciousness and settle the mind.
5. Mindfulness practice: This is contraindicated if it opens up the person too much, but it can be helpful for supporting the observing portion of the person's ego (or witness consciousness). This also may involve a strengthening of the person's connection to her or his basic sanity and ground of awareness. Except for those for whom mindfulness practice was a precipitating factor, this may be a very helpful practice.

Again, all meditation practices should be monitored very closely, and in many instances it is best to stop all meditation practices and eliminate entirely this kind of stimulation or activation, at least for a specific period of time.

SUMMARY

When spiritual emergency is supported and allowed to run its course, it moves the person toward an increasingly spiritual orientation. From an integral perspective, this can be part of a psychic shift in which the evolving soul or psychic center becomes a stronger influence in a person's life. It is the soul in us, the psychic entity, that, from behind the veil, shapes our life and draws us inexorably toward the inner depths and spiritual ground. This is a long process, involving many lifetimes, according to integral yoga, and sometimes the surface self needs a powerful reminder about what is important.

Spiritual emergency, for all of its destabilizing effects and disorganizing appearances, is a wake-up call. It is as if the inner being grabs the person by both lapels and shakes him or her, demanding that the surface self pay attention. To heal the fragmenting structures of the surface self and to bring about greater integration and cohesion is one goal of treatment. But for an integral psychotherapy, including this with a more spiritualized living and orientation is the optimal outcome. If the voice of the soul can be strengthened, if the impediments of the surface self to this deeper voice can be even partially cleared away, then there is a true resolution of spiritual emergency.

Notes

Chapter 1

1. Sri Aurobindo describes several other planes above our normal mentality that are superconscious and beyond current evolutionary awareness. These are the higher mind (where the Self has its native home), the illumined mind (where cognition is no longer of thought but of light), the intuitive mind (which approaches knowledge by identity), the overmind (the realm of the gods), and the supramental level (or pure truth consciousness).

Aurobindo describes the higher mind as "still very much on the mind level, although highly spiritual in its essential substance; and its instrumentation is through an elevated thought-power and comprehensive mental sight—not illumined by any of the intenser upper lights but as if in a large strong and clear daylight" (1978, p. 49).

The illumined mind is described as "a mind no longer of higher thought, but of spiritual light. Here the clarity of the spiritual intelligence, its tranquil daylight, gives place or subordinates itself to an intense lustre, a splendour and illumination of the Spirit: a play of lightnings of spiritual truth and power breaks from above into the consciousness and adds to the calm and wide enlightenment and the vast descent of peace which characterise or accompany the action of the larger conceptual-spiritual principle, a fiery ardour of realisation and rapturous ecstasy of knowledge. A downpour of inwardly visible light very usually envelopes this action" (1970, p. 944).

The higher mind and the illumined mind "enjoy their authority and can get their own united completeness only by a reference to a third level; for it is from the higher summits where dwells the intuitional being that they derive the knowledge which they turn into thought or sight and bring down to us for the mind's transmutation. Intuition is a power of consciousness nearer and more intimate to the original knowledge by identity; for it is always something that leaps out direct from a concealed identity. It is when the consciousness of the subject meets with the consciousness of the object, penetrates it and sees, feels or vibrates with the truth of what it contacts, that the intuition leaps out like a spark or lightning-flash from the shock of the meeting; or when the consciousness, even without any such meeting, looks into itself and feels directly and intimately the truth or the truths that are there or so contacts the hidden forces behind appearances, then also there is the outbreak of an intuitive light; . . . This close perception is more than sight, more than conception: it is the result of a penetrating and revealing touch which carries in it sight and conception as part of itself or as its natural consequence" (1970, pp. 946–947).

The Overmind is the last level before ascending to the supramental. "The consciousness . . . is experienced as a consciousness of Light and Truth, a power, force, action full of Light and Truth, an aesthesis and sensation of beauty and delight universal and multitudinous in detail, an illumination in the whole and in all things, in the one movement and all movements, with a constant extension and play of possibilities which is infinite. . . . All spiritual experiences are taken up and become normal to the new nature; all essential experiences belonging to the mind, life, body are taken up and spiritualized, transmuted and felt as forms of the consciousness, delight, power of the infinite existence. Intuition, illumined sight and thought enlarge themselves; their substance assumes a greater substantiality, mass, energy, their movement is more comprehensive, global, many-faceted, more wide and potent in its truth-force: the whole nature, knowledge, aesthesis, sympathy, feeling, dynamism become more catholic, all-understanding, all-embracing, cosmic, infinite" (1970, p. 952).

The supramental is the highest human power that is now seeking to manifest on earth. "Because its very nature is knowledge, it has not to acquire knowledge but possesses it in its own right; its steps are not from . . . ignorance to some imperfect light, but from truth to greater truth, from right perception to deeper perception, from intuition to intuition, from illumination to utter and boundless luminousness, from growing widenesses to the utter vasts and to very infinitude. . . . It starts from truth and light and moves always in truth and light" (1978, p. 157).

Thus there is a *horizontal* dimension of depth to consciousness (outer being, inner being, true being, psychic being) and a *vertical* dimension of height to consciousness (body-heart-mind leading to the higher mind planes).

Aurobindo describes these two dimensions of consciousness in this way:

There are in fact two systems simultaneously active in the organisation of the being and its parts: one is concentric, a series of rings or sheaths with the psychic at the centre; another is vertical, an ascension and descent, like a flight of steps, a series of superimposed planes with the supermind-overmind as the crucial nodus of the transition beyond the human into the Divine. For this transition, if it is to be at the same time a transformation, there is only one way, one path. First, there must be a conversion inwards, a going within to find the inmost psychic being and bring it out to the front, disclosing at the same time the inner mind, inner vital, inner physical parts of the nature. Next, there must be an ascension, a series of conversions upwards and a turning down to convert the lower parts. When one has made the inward conversion, one psychicises the whole lower nature so as to make it ready for the divine change. Going upwards, one passes beyond the human mind and at each stage of the ascent, there is a new conversion into a new consciousness into the whole of the nature. Thus rising beyond intellect through illuminated higher mind to the intuitive consciousness, we begin to look at everything not from the intellect range or through intellect as an instrument, but from a greater intuitive height and through an intuitivised will, feeling, emotion, sensation and physical contact. So, proceeding from Intuition to a greater overmind height, there is a new conversion and we look at and experience everything from the overmind consciousness and through a mind, heart, vital and body surcharged with the overmind thought, sight, will, feeling, sensation, play of force and contact. But the last conversion is the supramental, for once there—once the nature is supramentalised, we are beyond the Ignorance and conversion of consciousness is no longer needed, though a farther divine progression, even an infinite development is still possible. (1978, p. 251)

2. The two most ambitious attempts to construct an inclusive, psycho-spiritual model, by Wilber and Grof, have been good first efforts but are deficient in several respects. Wilber's model fails on two major counts, psychological and spiritual. First, Wilber (1986, 2000) places different psychologies and psychotherapies in a developmental line based on degree of integration. This betrays a fundamental misunderstanding of psychotherapy systems. By linking psychoanalysis to clients with "prepersonal level issues" (e.g., borderline, neurotic) and humanistic and existential therapies to clients with more integrated, "personal" level issues, Wilber places different systems at different levels of personality integration. But psychoanalysis and existential therapies deal extensively with clients at all levels of personality integration. In fact, it was existential therapy that pioneered innovative approaches to psychosis (Laing, 1965, 1967). Classifying schools of psychology according to degrees of personality integration is not a workable scheme.

Second, the nontheistic, Impersonal Divine bias of Wilber's model is an inadequate accounting of spiritual experience from an integral perspective. By denigrating the Personal Divine dimension of the spiritual picture, it privileges the dimension of the Impersonal Divine and unfortunately perpetuates Buddhist and *kevela advaita* claims to superiority, even as it claims to reconcile the theistic dimension of spiritual experience. Wilber's misinterpretation of Sri Aurobindo's integral philosophy would have Sri Aurobindo saying the exact opposite of what, in fact, he does say about the Personal and Impersonal Divine and, additionally, entirely distorts Sri Aurobindo's map of consciousness. (Parenthetically, the spiritual portion of Wilber's model also is based on several fictions about spiritual experience. Spiritual history demonstrates that spiritual realization does not unfold in the order that Wilber predicts and can even unfold in the opposite order that his model demands. As Aurobindo shows by personal example, the realization of the Impersonal Divine can come first, followed by the Personal Divine, followed by the intermediate zone or subtle plane realizations. This falsifies Wilber's claim to a universal order and developmental sequence.) Both the psychological and the spiritual parts of this psycho-spiritual model are untenable.

Grof's model falls short on several fronts. Grof (1975, 2000) tries a modified and more sophisticated version of Wilber's strategy in his attempt to integrate systems of psychotherapy. He places systems of psychology and psychotherapy in a linear hierarchy based on depth of consciousness. He places psychoanalysis on the most superficial layer to explain biographical psychology, then gestalt and Reichian psychology, which he believes represent deeper psychological experience, followed by his perinatal layers of birth trauma, followed by Jungian psychology in the deepest archetypal and transpersonal realms. This is unsatisfactory for several reasons. First, to say one type of depth psychology is "deeper" than another is problematic. Psychoanalysis can be as deep or deeper than gestalt, which also can be quite superficial depending as much upon the therapist as the theory. Degree of depth (Grof) is equally unworkable as degree of integration (Wilber).

Second, Grof does not account for contemporary psychoanalysis and intersubjectivity, or their many variations and schools, only the classical roots of psychoanalysis from a half century ago. This leaves out most of Western depth psychology. Third, perinatal material, Grof's biggest discovery, may have a far smaller impact upon development and psychology than he proposes. Fourth, psychological discoveries derived from work with altered states of consciousness, while intense and powerful at the time, have questionable value when generalized to cover the entire psyche when it is not in an altered state. The spiritual literature amply documents that a perspective that is true in one state of consciousness may be irrelevant or untrue in another state of consciousness. Clinical experience reinforces this view, for although some improvement of symptoms may occur in altered states, a complete working through does not appear to happen with his "nonordinary states" therapy (see Cortright, 1997, for a fuller discussion of these issues).

3. In Tibetan Buddhism, the psychic center is called the *tigl*, though it is subordinated to Buddha-nature in this tradition.

CHAPTER 2

1. The Vedas, the most ancient sacred texts that form the basis of Vedanta, were composed thousands of years ago for a much earlier mentality than that of the modern world. Symbolism and poetic metaphor abound in these archaic texts, making them difficult for the modern mind to penetrate, yet they contain a depth of spiritual wisdom that forms the basis of Hinduism today. The Vedas contain a great number of hymns devoted to Agni, the first of the Powers, first before all of the other gods. Sri Aurobindo believed that the Vedic hymns to Agni represent hymns to the psychic center with its force and light. Agni is variously imaged as the fire and flaming will of the Divine, as a Truth-Conscious soul, a seer, as the priest of the sacrifice whose mission is to purify and raise up the struggling aspirant to the light.

> The Veda speaks of the divine Flame in a series of splendid and opulent images. He is the rapturous priest of the sacrifice, the God-Will intoxicated with its own delight, the young sage, the sleepless envoy, the ever-wakeful flame in the house, the master of our gated dwelling-place, the beloved guest, the lord in the creature, the seer of the flaming tresses, the divine child, the pure and virgin God, the invincible warrior, the leader on the path who marches in front of the human peoples, the immortal in mortals, the worker established in man by the gods, the unobstructed in knowledge, the infinite

in being, the vast and flaming sun of the Truth, . . . the divine perception, the light, the vision. . . . Throughout the Veda it is in the hymns which celebrate this strong and brilliant deity that we find those which are the most splendid in poetic colouring, profound in psychological suggestion and sublime in their mystic intoxication. (Aurobindo, 1971b, p. 361)

Agni is interpreted by Aurobindo as the ancient symbol for the psychic center and its power, for it is this light that each person must awaken so that it can illumine life's path. Agni also is a force for purification that burns away the dross of our dense nature and purifies our outer being. Agni protects against the demons that try to wreak havoc upon the world and humanity. The psychic center, Agni, is the leader of the evolution, the guide that shows us the way, a portion of the Divine that has within it an inherent truth sense and discernment.

For the sake of completeness it should be noted that there are many different experiences of inner fire. There is the fire of tapas (spiritual discipline and will), the fire of kundalini (the sleeping spiritual energy at the base of the spine), the fire and light from the illumined mind, and the fire of sexual passion and energy. Each of these experiences must be differentiated from the fire of Agni or the psychic fire. To light the psychic fire in the heart is the goal of integral psychology.

Perhaps a more modern symbol than fire is the electric light. The growing light of the psychic center can be imaged as a dimmer switch or rheostat in which the psychic light is very faint to begin with but with aspiration, meditation, and surrender it becomes brighter and brighter. Electric light is a more accurate image in some ways, because it is a steady and continuous light that does not flicker and vary in its intensity like a flame does. The psychic light is a steady light burning deep within the heart.

2. The reason the self disappears in enlightenment or transcendence is not because it never existed and was always an illusion, as the Buddhists and *advaitins* have argued, but because its utility is over. When the psychic center has developed far enough, it can emerge fully and take its place as the individualized spiritual being that is part of the central being—atman or Buddha-nature. The function of the ego is no longer necessary, for there is a new organizing principle at work, a spiritual and no longer strictly organismic principle, though the soul can fully use its organismic instruments. The ego functions remain (e.g., memory, orientation in time and space, coordination, integration of sensory and emotional experience, planning, reality testing, etc.), indeed, are necessary to function in the world. But the ego sense or separate "I" feeling disappears when its usefulness ends. Individuality remains while the ego dissolves. This individuality is the flowering of our long path of individuation, pursued through many incarnations, many cultures, and many historical epochs.

CHAPTER 3

1. It should be noted that *some* psychological healing can come via meditation and spiritual practice, but such healing tends to be haphazard and is not as comprehensive or thoroughgoing as is depth psychotherapy.

2. It is difficult to know if the emotional wounding at other times in human history was similar to or different from what we experience now, because we can only infer what the state of consciousness evolution was in earlier epochs. We do know, however, that there has been a historical development in how children are viewed. Up until the last century or two, children were viewed as small adults. The creation of child labor laws signaled a change in society's views of childhood.

When more empathic attention is given to children, a more fully developed self emerges, which is an expression of the evolution of consciousness. With changing family patterns and child-rearing practices, the development of the self changes as well. Today's core wounding occurs in the historical and cultural context of nuclear or extended families where childhood, adolescence, and adulthood are seen as distinct developmental phases. Attachment patterns to parents and siblings are crucial in considering wounding and the self's development.

3. The original meaning of the word "sin" is "to miss the mark," to not shoot straight or be off the mark. This is precisely the effect our defenses have on us. Because of our neurotic distortions, we do not perceive clearly, nor do we respond truly. Our defensive twists and contortions prevent us from shooting straight, and we end up missing the mark, or "sinning."

The Christian concept of "original sin" contends that every human being is born into a state of sin, and that this inheres in the human condition. Feeling that we are inherently bad, that something is intrinsically wrong with us, is this not the essence of the narcissistic wound? We do not know what it is or what we did, but narcissistic wounding casts a shadow over the self—feeling not okay, not all there, shameful, like something is wrong in the very core of our being. The narcissistic wound from our family of origin leaves an indelible imprint until healed. Would "original wound" be a more accurate concept than "original sin" to describe this basic human experience? But this would be to fall into the same reductionistic trap that psychology has fallen into all along when attempting to understand spiritual experience. For all of this, while true, does not entirely cover or explain "original sin." From an integral perspective, original sin began with the plunge into matter as spirit passed into a swoon of unconsciousness. The separation from spirit is the source of our existential pain, just as being separated from our soul and the Divine also causes us to miss the mark and "sin" as well. There is a psychological as well as a spiritual dimension to these notions. A psychological perspective clarifies how what are usually considered purely spiritual concepts may often be better described as psycho-spiritual.

4. Wounding is an extraordinarily complex phenomenon. It occurs many, many times in the course of development, at all levels of intensity and depth. There are layers and layers of defenses against this wounding that generally require years or even decades of working through. This discussion considers wounding in a global way as it affects all levels of the self. Each level has immense subtlety and complexity to it and to the defensive structures around it.

Now that psychological wounding has been placed in the larger context of the depth dimensions of the psyche, the following, four-level model of consciousness can be tentatively advanced:

	Conscious self (mix of authentic self with false self)
Outer Being	Defenses and unconscious shielding
(frontal self;	Impasse (existential void; hole; non-being)
body-heart-mind;	Core wounding
organism)	Authentic self's potential

- -

	Collective unconscious
Inner Being	Inner mind
	Inner vital
	Inner or subtle body (energy body; chakras)

- -

	True mind
True eing	True heart
	True physical

- -

	Psychic center (true soul)
Psychic Being	
(with atman and	
overhead planes above)	

Conventional Western psychology charts only the outer being, the frontal physi-cal-emotional-mental organism with which the self identifiesh. Jungian psychology, psychosynthesis, Ali's diamond school, and other transpersonal approaches go beyond traditional Western maps to include portions of inner being, but Eastern psychology excels at precisely charting the three inner levels of being.

The conscious self is a mixture of the true self, primary and compensatory struc-tures, on the one hand, and the false self, or defensive structures, on the other. What is authentic and what is inauthentic can only be known retrospectively, after successful psychotherapy allows the false self images and structures to fall away. Before that, inau-thentic patterns created from the defensive structures below are designed to cover, hide, and compensate for the loss of key energies and aspects of the self. For example, wounding around early dependency may by patched over with a defensive covering of independence and an outward denial of neediness, or it may result in dependent clingi-ness. Similarly, failure in affirming the nascent authentic self can result in low self-esteem and/or a covering of (false) grandiosity to hide the "bad" self.

Because of this amalgam of the authentic and inauthentic self, the conscious self tends, on the one hand, to be highly role-bound, operating from repetitive patterns that keep it safely away from threatening situations and feelings, using inauthentic ways of relating that reinforce these defensive structures. As these patterns and neural networks are reinforced and strengthened, real change becomes more difficult. On the other hand, there are areas where the conscious self is creative and spontaneous. These rela-tively conflict-free areas of the self are able to expand as the self becomes more inte-grated and more fully connected to its depths.

Below the conscious self are many layers of defenses. The earlier simplified chart does not reveal the many layers of defensive shielding that exist and slowly get worked through in depth psychotherapy ("peeling the onion"). However, it should be noted that defenses such as disavowal, repression, and dissociation are themselves multilayered. As the defenses gradually erode in psychotherapy, or at times of fragmentation and stress, the impasse layer is revealed. Here the gestalt term *impasse* is used, called the hole in Ali's approach, or the void in existentialism, a state of deficiency or empty nothingness. This is not the full, rich void of spiritual experience but an empty, deficient void of insufficiency and isolation, a cover for the wounded self and a first move away from the authentic self's potentials. It is like a scab that covers the wounded self but is itself a kind of non-being. It is also multilayered, with first experiences of this state of deficiency oftentimes resonating with more recent life experiences, for example of the 20s or 30s, then, going deeper, revealing periods in the person's teens of rejection, isolation, and shame, leading to earlier layers of this experience in latency and early childhood. This zone of empty deadness is difficult to tolerate, because it is a state of loss of the authentic self, of its abilities and potentials, and it is generally avoided.

It also appears in states of fragmentation, when we experience failure in work or relationships or blows to self-esteem. More often we try to escape from feeling this through coping strategies and inauthentic ways of being designed to cover up such shameful feelings. However, in tolerating and exploring this, it gradually melts away to reveal the core wounding from earliest childhood and such shame-laden feelings as badness, unworthiness, inadequacy, isolation, and alienation (literally feeling at times "like an alien"), a depressed, depleted experience of self.

When deep, experiential exploration of this vulnerable, hurt self occurs, there can be a healing of these early wounds and an emergence of the authentic self that lies beneath these early wounds. That is, when the core wounding is fully felt, expressed, worked through from first one side, then another, and then another, this wounding is cleansed and healed, and it moves forward as it gives way to the energies and potentials of the authentic self. This nucleus of possibilities, however, does not emerge fully grown but undergoes a slow developmental period of growth and modification that requires being welcomed and lovingly invited to come forth via nourishing, safe relationship(s).

The outermost layer of the inner being is the collective unconscious, discovered by Jung, with the archetypes as universal organizing principles. Integral psychology differentiates three aspects to the inner being—the inner mind, which is much larger and more powerful than the surface mind, more open to the universal forces of the cosmic mind; the inner heart or vital, which is aware of other forces, beings, and the universal impulses and forces of the intermediate plane; and the inner or subtle physical, consisting of the auric field, the chakras, and what is sometimes called the energy body.

The third level consists of the true being, the true mental, true emotional, true physical being. This appears to be what Jung referred to as the Self and what Ali calls "essence." It is a source of non-egoic, spiritual qualities and represents the atman on each plane. Because it relates to the atman, an exceedingly difficult realization, it is difficult to remain in the state of the true being for very long. These intervening layers of the inner being and true being may or may not become conscious as the psychic center awakens, or, more commonly, they may become conscious without the psychic center awakening.

The fourth level is the psychic being, with the atman and overhead planes above. The true soul or psychic center is the inmost core of our being, the secret foundation of psychological life, as it puts forth a new outer being (*svabhava*) each lifetime that expresses its authentic nature. A pure flame of aspiration and bhakti for the divine, the psychic center is the evolutionary element within us, progressing ceaselessly until it achieves union with the Divine. This radiant center of love and wisdom is our one infallible source of guidance, a discriminating intelligence whose influence we need to cultivate to discover our life path.

CHAPTER 4

1. Traditional evolutionary psychology considers only our animal past to understand motivation. Integral evolutionary psychology also includes our spiritual future in assessing the forces acting upon the psyche in its developmental trajectory.

2. Another casualty of postmodernism is the entire concept of authenticity. This is a logical outcome of its denial of the depths. From postmodernism's surface view, if all positions and perspectives have validity, then authenticity itself becomes impossible, for how can one part be more authentically me than any other part? However, when we discover our depths, we find that some aspects of our experience are indeed more truly and authentically who we are, while other, more surface feelings, behaviors, or images are but masks designed to cover over certain feelings and are to that degree inauthentic. Authenticity inheres in a psychology of the depths.

3. Aurobindo goes beyond to describe two further transformations: the spiritual and the supramental. The spiritual transformation brings down the spirit's power and light from above, and the supramental transformation ends in a perfect spiritualized, truth-consciousness that transforms the very cells of the body itself. These are far away from most people, whereas the psychological and psychic transformations that are the focus of this book are within reach of all sincere aspirants.

CHAPTER 7

1. Sri Ramanuja has seven types of practice for the development of bhakti. These are:

  1. *Viveka*—the practice of discrimination, being careful what we take into our system through the senses. Particular attention is given to food, so that only purity-generating and *sattwic* (peace-giving) food is eaten, prepared by people and conditions that are pure.
  2. *Vimoka*—resisting passions such as anger, sexuality, and jealousy.
  3. *Abhyasa*—practices such as worship, devotional singing, and visiting holy places on pilgrimages.
  4. *Kriya*—the fivefold duties of life. These include duties toward divine spirits and angels through rituals, duty to spiritual teachers through reading sacred texts and literature, duty to ancestors, and duty to nature (an ecological awareness that explicitly affirms that animals and plants as part of God's

creation and are not to be destroyed or exploited) through cultivating an attitude of harmony.

5. *Kalyana*—practicing virtues such as truth (*satya*), kindness, straightforward-ness, love of all beings, and non-harming (*ahimsa*).

6. *Anavasada*—keeping a cheerful and positive attitude, free from despair and pessimism.

7. *Anuddharsa*—equality, not yielding to depression or excitement.

Other examples of bhakti yoga include the ninefold discipline from the *Bhagavat Purana*. These are:

- hearing about God's majesty
- singing His praise with others (devotional singing, chanting)
- mantra, or silent remembrance of God through repetition of his names
- worship of holy images
- saluting His presence in all beings
- cultivating an attitude of servantship
- service to God in His aspect of society
- entertaining intimacy with Him
- making a wholehearted and an unreserved offering to Him

From the stream of Sri Nimbarka's tradition of *dvaitadvaita* (duality in unity) comes the following six precepts:

1. Cherish love for all, for all beings constitute God's body
2. Abstain from evil to all and hostility to Him
3. Faith, that God will protect the devotee
4. Choosing God as one's shelter
5. Entrusting oneself to Him
6. Humbleness, absence of pride, readiness to accept misfortune, and failure as the Divine will

Other examples could be given, but it becomes clear that all schools of bhakti yoga have roughly similar principles and practices.

2. The psychological work of opening the heart is to allow the full force of emo-tion to flow freely. Thus work with anger, for example, aims not just at completing unfinished anger from the past but at letting anger flow without obstruction, in all ranges and intensities, so it may organize our actions and complete its purpose. Our skill at expressing anger increases with practice.

Anger is not bottomless, as many spiritual traditions assert, nor is it a meaningless sign of sin or impurity. It has a meaning and an essential purpose in living. But to make sense of its energy and action we must get to its roots. For this it is necessary to go all the way, to encounter the full depths of violence, resentment, and rage that live in the human psyche. Only in making the journey into the underworld and thoroughly plumbing these depths can we find the redeeming light hidden in these dark recesses and make it available for our life.

The cultural fear of anger is understandable, for repressed anger can erupt in uncontrolled and destructive ways. Seeing rage-prone people and some borderline personality disorders who seem helpless in the grip of anger further reinforces this fear (and living with such unrestrained, out-of-control anger also has serious health consequences, such as high cholesterol, atherosclerosis, high incidence of heart attacks, etc.). Yet the "rage-aholic" is hardly the model of skill at relating to anger, merely the dark, flip side of our cultural aversion to it.

The research evidence on anger is confused and contradictory in how to best work with anger. Since many researchers are not trained in depth psychology, the questions asked and the measures used will oftentimes confound the results. Clearly some people only get angrier in doing cathartic expression, but here the self structure of the person must be considered. If the person is borderline or rage-prone, until the underlying personality structure becomes more cohesive and the real roots of rage-proneness are discovered, then mere catharsis will be ineffective and will perpetuate poor impulse control. On the other hand, catharsis can be very helpful for overly constrained, constricted, neurotic clients who inhibit the expression of anger.

Working with and resolving excessive anger can take many forms depending upon the personality organization of the person, the family history, emotional intelligence, and resilience. For most people it is a matter of unflinchingly, courageously opening up to these energies, fully feeling and exploring them so that rather than being controlled by them they can truly master these powerful life energies.

As anger is owned and its guidance incorporated into daily life, and as the influence of the psychic center grows, working with anger can become a psycho-spiritual practice. Expressing our anger authentically *and* compassionately becomes a way of honoring anger's wisdom and the soul's love. Truth in the context of compassion is the goal—neither suppressing nor denying anger out of a spiritual "should," nor indulging in anger in a destructive way. Speaking our truth in a loving way that is both clear and direct as well as respectful and loving is a challenge that takes us to another level in relating to anger (see Cortright, Kahn, and Hess, 2003, for a fuller discussion).

CHAPTER 8

1. While such stopgap measures may be useful for reducing stress in the short run, by focusing on symptom removal rather than working with the underlying causes this approach works well as a Band-Aid but does not address the larger, depth psychological issues that have created the problem in the first place. Further, it is not clear which level of the heart is being referred to in these studies. While the physical heart is what is being measured in most of this literature, from an integral perspective this is just the most outward, material level of the heart. Some of what occurs in this research may in fact be tapping into the heart chakra and the feelings from this deeper, subtle heart within, but the published research seems to conflate the different levels of the heart.

2. In awakening our body consciousness there are several points of approach. Simple mindfulness is the most direct and powerful discipline for reinhabiting our physical being. Becoming aware of our physicality and sensuality means really paying

attention to the joy inherent in embodied living. Whether showering, walking along
the street, looking at the world, reaching for a book on a shelf, or talking to a friend,
our world abounds with sensory wonders. Charlotte Selver's groundbreaking work with
"sensory awareness" stands as one of the great developments in the human potential
movement. Her work influenced a couple of generations of somatic and existential
therapists.

A second point of approach involves healing the emotional dissociation from the
body. This was Wilhelm Reich's great insight into how defending against emotional
wounding involves a flight into the mind and out of the body. All of the humanistic,
existential, and somatic therapies derive from this fundamental understanding, and
focusing is perhaps the essential attentional skill needed to heal dissociation. All body-
oriented therapies, including gestalt, bioenergetics, Hakomi, breathwork, Reichian
therapy, core energetics, bodynamics, and existential therapy, bring consciousness back
into the body and attend to physical sensations and the breath, and all are useful in an
integral approach to psychotherapy, for all help bring the right hemisphere more fully
on-line.

A third point of approach is through improving physical health. This involves
many different disciplines. Although not a substitute for therapeutic working through,
physical exercise, when done consciously and with the aspiration for deepening somatic
awareness, is one of the best means for improving mental alertness, emotional well-
being, and physical health. The West has excelled in the development of physical exercise for the outer body, from muscle fitness, strength, and endurance, to aerobic
training. The East has excelled in the development of subtle physical exercise that
draws the vital energy from the subtle physical body into the outer, physical body
through such disciplines as yoga, tai chi, qi gong, and aikido. Together, Western (yang
approaches) and Eastern (yin approaches), or physical and subtle physical, exercises
bring new vitality and aliveness to our physical being and bring out the energetic, subtle
substratum underlying our body.

Bodywork and subtle bodywork are further means to improve physical health.
Bodywork such as Rolfing, Feldenkrais, massage, osteopathy, cranial-sacral work, and,
of course, Western medicine offers immense new possibilities for improving health.
Subtle bodywork, such as acupuncture, homeopathy, Reiki, and energy work, can work
with the subtle physical or energy body and correct imbalances that can later result in
disease.

Diet is a significant factor in health, and an integral approach must take into
account a number of factors:

- the type of food a person eats (balance of protein, fat, carbohydrate; type of
  fats; quality of protein and carbohydrate; how cooked, etc.)
- the supplements taken
- the drugs consumed in eating (caffeine, chocolate, theobromine)
- the amount of food eaten
- the consciousness put into the preparation (by cooks, etc.)
- the consciousness of eating itself

Eating too much reduces consciousness; eating overly stimulating foods or stimulants
or certain supplements can produce central nervous system stimulation that takes a

person away from the heart and into the mind; some foods and supplements stimulate the outer consciousness and reduce awareness of the inner consciousness; eating for emotional reasons becomes a way to regulate affect and diminish awareness; the act of eating itself is generally fairly unconscious, as is the energy put into the food during preparation. All of these factors figure into how food affects consciousness.

Strengthening the immune system occurs both through attending to the afore-mentioned elements and working through the emotional wounding and defenses. The testimony from a number of individuals who are sensitive to subtle energy fields is that emotional difficulties have a significant impact upon the subtle body and the auric field (Brennan, 1987, 1993; Myss, 1988, 1996). These distortions in the subtle body eventu-ally cause disease or breakdown in the physical body. Improving emotional well-being, on the other hand, not only positively affects the energy field, but it also directly improves the immune system (Pert, 1997, 1998). Improving one's immune system and overall health and vitality has the side effect of enhancing mood, energy, and emotional well-being.

Beyond these techniques and practices, it is the aspiration to awaken the body that draws to us people, teachers, books, and experiences that aid in this process. As the body awakens and consciousness deepens into the inner ranges of physical being, there is a spontaneous opening up to these inner energies that will gradually refine the body. Refinement brings a greater sensitivity and lightness to the body, a greater responsive-ness to subtle physical, psychic, and spiritual forces. It is not that a refined body is skinny and a dense body is fat; refinement implies nothing about the outer form or shape of the body. Rather, refinement pertains to the quality of the substance of the body. As the body awakens and refines, new levels of awareness develop, and the mir-acle of embodiment reveals higher and deeper ranges of bliss, energy, vitality, light, and harmony that become the new ground of our physical existence.

3. In discussing the psychic center or evolving soul, it is inevitable that some will mistake their own limited experiences for the true thing. Already in the spiritual marketplace there are self-proclaimed "spiritual teachers" who assert that they have realized their psychic being and are helping their students do the same. However, to one who has some degree of psychic realization, it is quite obvious through these teach-ers' words and actions that such assertions are the result of ego inflation and self-decep-tion. The Mother counsels that if there is any doubt about whether an experience is the psychic being, it is not. However, surety does not provide immunity from self-decep-tion. The power of unconscious narcissism is great, and the lure of becoming a great yogi or spiritual teacher is one of the first hazards encountered.

4. It has long been an article of faith in depth therapy (originally asserted by Freud) that a client's desire to get better is not sufficient motivation to fully engage psychotherapy. Therefore, it is necessary to use the transference so the client will get better in order to please the therapist. Integral psychotherapy challenges this assump-tion and finds it an inadequate understanding of human motivation. It is an infan-tilizing belief that derives from the psychoanalytic frame of reference and overlooks the soul's inherent drive for growth and fulfillment. Integral psychotherapy reverses this so that pleasing the therapist is secondary, and the client's aspiration for whole-ness is primary.

APPENDIX A

1. Each of these different schools of Indian philosophy represents a certain spiritual experience, a certain status of consciousness. The experiences of the founders of these schools became enthroned as the highest, and in the philosophical elaborations that followed, all other spiritual realizations were then given a lower ranking. It is rare to find a mature soul so well rounded and developed as to have extensive experience of the full range of spiritual realizations. Sri Ramakrishna, a leading figure in the Indian cultural renaissance in the late 19th century, was just such a master soul whose great spiritual power helped galvanize Indian spirituality and sowed the seeds for an integration of the different wisdom traditions of the world. But Ramakrishna was not destined to provide a philosophical basis or to give an intellectual expression to this depth of spiritual realization. This was to be the task of Sri Aurobindo, a spiritual culminating point in Indian philosophy.

2. *Kevala advaita* is right when it importantly stresses the reality of Brahman, its formless, indeterminable, static aspect of *nirguna* and its impersonal nature. Yet it is limited by admitting no other sides of Brahman into the picture. It errs in putting all qualities, all differentiations of the universe, and the personal dimension of Brahman into the category of illusion and dismissing them. This produces the unfortunate result of world negation, where asceticism and self-denial are idealized as life and the material plane is abandoned.

Visistadvaita and the related schools of *suddhadvaita*, *dvaitadvaita*, and *advaya* are correct in pointing to the personal nature of the Divine, *saguna* Brahman, and the bountiful qualities and attributes inherent in Brahman. They rightly stress the reality of the world and the individual soul, but they limit themselves in relegating the impersonal, static dimension of Brahman to a secondary status.

Dvaita importantly affirms the reality of the world and the reality of differentiation. But its insistence upon the eternal relation of difference between souls and Brahman is a one-sided view of liberation, and it underemphasizes the spiritual possibility of merging into the transcendent Ground.

Tantra goes farther in affirming the reality of existence, and its technique of a spiritual conquest of embodied life is preferable to a world-negating escape. Tantra's charting of the subtle energy realm, the chakra system, and the kundalini process, along with its focus on the Shakti or Divine Mother dimension, is essential to a complete spirituality. But even here the method leads to a liberation from material life and an eventual escape from the round of birth and death. With its focus on physical and subtle physical energies in its practices it easily slips into a kind of subtle materialistic reductionism that can ignore the central spiritual contributions of heart and mind by concentrating instead on the energy body and the raising of kundalini energy up the spine.

3. When the vital principle of Life manifested, it took up the physical level and transformed it into something new: living cells that have different properties than inanimate matter. When Mind emerged out of Life, it further transformed matter: animal

tissue is different from plant tissue. Each new level as it emerged turned its powers on what came before it to produce an evolutionary shift in the previous levels.

In human beings, with the full emergence of mind, this process takes yet another step forward. We see the results of this already, as mind now consciously turns its powers on the evolutionary process. On the physical level, we have vastly improved nutrition, medicine, and health care, better physical training and conditioning, resulting in better athletic performance, and longer life. We now stand on the threshold of genetic manipulation that has the potential to further transform the physical level for the better (though also the danger of harming our physical foundation if used prematurely). Mind improves the heart level through such methods as emotional healing and psychotherapy, learning to relate to others more fully and lovingly, and more knowledgeable and emotionally attuned child-rearing practices that result in less wounded, more emotionally healthy adults. Mind improves its own level through better education, new knowledge, new ways of learning, and neurally stimulating environments, such as the Internet, computers, and cyberspace. As the spiritual transformation unfolds, it in turn will effect a change in the mind, the emotional, and the body in order to develop them even more fully and to better express the spiritual consciousness within.

4. Most spiritual traditions seek a heaven away from the earth plane, a spiritual beyond rather than a spiritualized existence here. The goal in the Impersonal paths is to merge into the oceanic consciousness of Brahman (or Buddha-nature or Tao), extinguish the ego, and pass out of the manifest existence. Since life is seen as a mirage or a pointless round of suffering, the best solution is to transcend it all and move into a beyond. Mahayana Buddhism holds out the boddhisattva ideal, where compassionate beings renounce enlightenment until all sentient beings achieve nirvana first. This is much closer to an integral approach, but even here life is seen as something to get beyond. To abandon the earth plane is still the goal, but compassion brings the helping hand of the boddhisattva, who has the good grace to say, "After you." Even most theistic conceptions see a heaven as the final salvation. Although most of the theistic traditions stress the reality of the world and the manifested universe, they also tend to ascribe a lower reality to the material plane and to place a higher value on a heavenly abode that is more perfect and eternal, the place of ultimate salvation.

References

Anon. (2001). *Katha Upanishad*. Translated by Swami Ambikananda. New York: Viking Studio.

Almaas, A. H. (1986). *Essence*. Berkeley, CA: Diamond Books.

Almaas, A. H. (1988). *Pearl beyond price*. Berkeley, CA: Diamond Books.

Almaas, A. H. (1996). *The point of existence*. Berkeley, CA: Diamond Books.

Aurobindo, Sri. (1970). *The life divine*. Pondicherry: Sri Aurobindo Ashram Press.

Aurobindo, Sri. (1971a). *Letters on yoga*. Pondicherry: Sri Aurobindo Ashram Press.

Aurobindo, Sri. (1971b). *The secret of the veda*. Pondicherry: Sri Aurobindo Ashram Press.

Aurobindo, Sri. (1972). *Essays on the gita*. Pondicherry: Sri Aurobindo Ashram Press.

Aurobindo, Sri. (1972b). *On himself*. Pondicherry: Sri Aurobindo Ashram Press.

Aurobindo, Sri. (1973a). *The supramental manifestation upon earth*. Pondicherry: Sri Aurobindo Ashram Press.

Aurobindo, Sri (1973b). *Synthesis of yoga*. Pondicherry: Sri Aurobindo Ashram Press.

Aurobindo, Sri. (1977). *The human cycle*. Pondicherry: Sri Aurobindo Ashram Press.

Aurobindo, Sri. (1978). *Glossary of terms in Sri Aurobindo's writings*. Pondicherry: Sri Aurobindo Ashram Press.

Aurobindo, Sri. (1994). *Essays divine and human*. Pondicherry: Sri Aurobindo Ashram Press.

Basch, M. (1988). *Understanding psychotherapy*. New York: Basic Books.

Beck, A. (1979). *Cognitive therapy and the emotional disorders*. New York: Penguin Books.

Beck, A. (1985). *Anxiety disorders and phobias*. New York: Basic Books.

Beck, A. (1987). *Cognitive therapy of depression*. New York: Guilford Press.

Beebe, B., & Lachman, F. M. (1994). Representation and internalization in infancy: Three principles of salience. *Psychoanalytic Psychology, 11*, 127–166.

Bogart, G. (1992). Separating from a spiritual teacher. *Journal of Transpersonal Psychology*, *24*(1), 1–22.

Brennan, B. (1987). *Hands of light*. New York: Bantam Books.

Brennan, B. (1993). *Light emerging*. New York: Bantam Books.

Broucsek, F. (1991). *Shame and the self*. New York: Guilford Press.

Bugental, J. (1978). *Psychotherapy and process*. Menlo Park, CA: Addison-Wesley.

Chaudhuri, H. (1973). *Sri Aurobindo: Prophet of the life divine*. San Francisco: Cultural Integration Fellowship.

Chaudhuri, H. (1974). *Being, evolution, and immortality*. Wheaton, IL: Theosophical Publishing House.

Chaudhuri, H. (1977). *The evolution of integral consciousness*. Wheaton, IL: Theosophical Publishing House.

Childre, D., & Martin, H. (1999). *The heartmath solution*. San Francisco: Harper San Francisco.

Chiron, C., Jambaque, I., Nabbout, R., Lounes, R., Syrota, A., & Dulac, O. (1997). The right brain hemisphere is dominant in human infants. *Brain, 120,* 1057–1065.

Cornelissen, M., & Joshi, K. (2004). *Consciousness, Indian psychology, and yoga*. New Delhi: Center for the Study of Civilizations.

Cortright, B. (1997). *Psychotherapy and spirit*. Albany: State University of New York Press.

Cortright, B., Kahn, M., & Hess, J. (2003). Speaking from the heart: Integral T-groups as a tool for training transpersonal psychotherapists. *The Journal of Transpersonal Psychology, 35* (2), 127–142.

Csikszentmihalyi, M. (1990). *Flow*. New York: Harper & Row.

Csikszentmihalyi, M. (1997). *Finding flow*. New York: Basic Books.

Cushman, P. (1995). *Constructing the self, constructing America*. Reading, MA: Addsion-Wesley.

Engler, J. (1986). Therapeutic aims in psychotherapy and meditation. In K. Wilber, J. Engler, & D. Brown, *Transformations of consciousness* (pp. 17–51) Boston: Shambhala.

Epstein, M. (1996). *Thoughts without a thinker*. New York: Basic Books.

Fairbairn, W. R. D. (1954). *An object relations theory of the personality*. New York: Basic Books.

Fonagy, P. (2001). *Attachment theory and psychoanalysis*. New York: Other Press.

Frager, R. (1999). *Heart, self, and soul*. Wheaton, Il: Theosophical Publishing House.

Gazzaniga, M. S. (1985). *The social brain: Discovering the networks of the mind*. New York: Basic Books.

Gendlin, E. (1981). *Focusing*. New York: Basic Books.

Gendlin, E. (1996). *Focusing-oriented psychotherapy*. New York: Guilford Press.

Gerard, R. (1988). Symbolic apperception and integral psychology. *Journal of Esoteric Psychology,4* (2), 95–1988.

Goleman, D. (1995). *Emotional intelligence*. New York: Bantam Books.

Goleman, D., & Gurin, J. (Eds.) (1993). *Mind/Body medicine*. New York: Consumer Reports.

Grandcolas, A. (2004). *The psychic being and the bursting of its veil* (Monograph). Auroville, India.

Grof, S. (1975). *Realms of the human unconscious*. New York: Viking Press.

Grof, S. (1985). *Beyond the brain*. Albany: State University of New York Press.

Grof, C., & Grof, S. (1989). *Spiritual emergency*. Los Angeles: Tarcher.

Grof, S. (2000). *Psychology of the future*. Albany: State University of New York Press.

Guntrip, H. (1969). *Schizoid phenomenon, object relations, and the self*. New York: International Universities Press.

Jacobson, E. (1964). *The self and the object world*. New York: International Universities Press.

Jung, C. (1975). *Letters Vol I*. p. 73 ed. Adler, G. Princeton: Princeton University Press.

Kabat-Zinn, J. (1990). *Full catastrophe living*. Surrey, England: Delta.

Kahn, M. (2002). *Basic Freud*. New York: Basic Books.

Kernberg, O. (1975). *Borderline conditions and pathological narcissism*. New York: Jason Aranson.

Kernberg, O. (1980). *Internal world and external reality*. New York: Jason Aronson.

Kipling, R. (1994). *The sayings of Rudyard Kipling*. London: Duckworth Publishing.

Klein, M. (1975a). *Envy and gratitude and other works*. New York: Dell.

Klein, M. (1975b). *Love, guilt, and reparation and other works*. New York: Dell.

Kohut, H. (1971). *The analysis of the self*. New York: International Universities Press.

Kohut, H. (1977). *The restoration of the self*. Madison, CT: International Universities Press.

Kohut, H. (1984). *How does analysis cure?* Chicago: University of Chicago Press.

Krishnamurti, J. (1958). *Commentaries on living*. Wheaton, IL: Quest.

Kuhn, T. (1970). *The structure of scientific revolutions*. Chicago: University of Chicago Press.

Kurtz, R. (1990). *Body-centered psychotherapy*. Mendocino, CA: Life Rhythm.

Laing, R. D. (1965). *The divided self*. Baltimore: Penguin.

Laing, R.D. (1967). *The politics of experience*. New York: Ballantine.

Lewis, T., Amini, F., & Lannon, R. (2000). *A general theory of love*. New York: Random House.

Linehan, M. (1993). *Cognitive-behavioral treatment of borderline personality disorder*. New York: Guilford.

Lowen, A. (1975). *Bioenergetics*. New York: Penguin Books.

Lukoff, D., & Everest, H. (1985). The myths in mental illness. *Journal of Transpersonal Psychology, 17*(2), 123–153.

Lukoff, D., Lu, F., & Turner, R. (1998). From spiritual emergency to spiritual problem. *Journal of Humanistic Psychology, 38*(2), 157–186.

Murphy, G. (1958). *Human potentialities*. New York: Basic Books.

Myss, C. (1988). *The creation of health*. New York: Three Rivers Press.

Myss, C. (1996). *Anatomy of the spirit*. New York: Three Rivers Press.

Nathanson, D. (1992). *Shame and pride*. New York: W. W. Norton & Co.

Nelson, J. (1990). *Healing the split*. Los Angeles: Tarcher.

Perls, F. (1969). *Gestalt therapy verbatim*. Moab, UT: Real People Press.

Perls, F., Hefferline, R., & Goodman, P. (1951). *Gestalt therapy*. New York: Dell Publishing Co.

Perry, J. (1953). *The self in psychotic process*. Berkeley: University of California Press.

Perry, J. (1976). *Roots of renewal in myth and madness*. San Francisco: Jossey-Bass.

Pert, C. (1997). *The molecules of emotion*. New York: Scribner.

Pert, C. (1998). The psychosomatic network: Foundations of mind-body medicine. *Alternative Therapies, 4*(4), 30–40.

Pierrakos, J. (1990). *Core energetics*. Mendocino, CA: Life Rhythm.

Richards, P., & Bergin, A. (1997). *A spiritual strategy for counseling and psychotherapy*. Washington, DC: American Psychological Association.

Rogers, C. (1961). *On becoming a person*. New York: Houghton Mifflin.

Ross, E. D., Homan, R. W., & Buck, R. (1994). Differential hemispheric lateralization of primary and social emotions. *Neuropsychiatry, Neuropsychology, and Behavioral Neurology, 7*, 1–19.

Rubin, J. (1996). *Psychotherapy and Buddhism*. New York: Plenum.

Russek, L., & Schwartz, G. (1994). Interpersonal heart-brain registration and the perception of parental love: A 42-year follow-up of the Harvard mastery-of-stress study. *Subtle Energies, 5*(3).

Sargeant, W. (1984). *Bhagavad gita*. Albany: State University of New York Press.

Saugstad, L. F. (1998). Cerebral lateralization and rate of maturation. *International Journal of Psychophysiology, 28*, 37–62.

Schore, A. (1999). *Affect regulation and the origin of the self.* Mahwah, NJ: Lawrence Erlbaum Associates.

Schore, A. (2003a). *Affect dysregulation and disorders of the self.* New York: Norton.

Schore, A. (2003b). *Affect regulation and the repair of the self.* New York: Norton.

Sen, I. (1986). *Integral psychology.* Pondicherry, India: Sri Aurobindo Ashram Press.

Sharma, C. (1964). *A critical survey of Indian philosophy.* Delhi: Motilal Banarsidass.

Siegel, D. (1999). *The developing mind.* New York: Guilford Press.

Smith, H. (1976). *Forgotten truth.* New York: HarperCollins.

Smith, H. (1982). *Beyond the postmodern mind.* Wheaton, IL: Theosophical Publishing House.

Song, L., Schwartz, G., & Russek, L. (1998). Heart-focused attention and heart-brain synchronization. *Alternative Therapies in Health and Medicine, 4*(5), 44–62.

Stolorow, R., Brandchaft, B., & Atwood, G. (1987). *Psychoanalytic treatment.* Hillsdale, NJ: The Analytic Press.

Stroufe, L. A., Egeland, B., & Kreutzer, T. (1990). The fate of early experience following childhood change: Longitudinal approaches to individual adaptation in childhood. *Child Development, 61,* 1363–1373.

Swami Prabhavananda, & Manchester, F. (Trans.). (1947). *The Upanishads: Breath of the eternal.* Hollywood, CA: Vedanta Press.

Tomkins, S. (1963). Affect/Imagery/Consciousness. In *The negative affects:* Vol. 2. New York: Springer.

Washburn, M. (1988). *The ego and the dynamic ground.* Albany: State University of New York Press.

Washburn, M. (1994). *Transpersonal psychology in psychoanalytic perspective.* Albany: State University of New York Press.

Wilber, K. (1986). *Transformations of consciousness.* Boston: Shambhala.

Wilber, K. (2000). *Integral psychology.* Boston: Shambhala.

Winnicott, D. W. (1958). *Collected papers: through pediatrics to psycho-analysis.* London: Tavistock.

Winnicott, D. W. (1965). *Maturational processes and the facilitating environment.* New York: International Universities Press.

Winnicott, D. W. (1971). *Playing and reality.* New York: Basic Books.

Wurmser, L. (1981). *The mask of shame.* Baltimore, MD: Johns Hopkins University Press.

Yalom, I. (1980). *Existential psychotherapy.* New York: Basic Books.

Index